Gastrointestinal Disorders and Nutrition

■ · · · · · · ■

Tonia Reinhard, M.S., R.D.

Contemporary Books

Chicago   New York   San Francisco   Lisbon   Madrid   Mexico City
Milan   New Delhi   San Juan   Seoul   Singapore   Sydney   Toronto

Library of Congress Cataloging-in-Publication Data

Reinhard, Tonia.
   Gastrointestinal disorders and nutrition / Tonia Reinhard.
      p. cm.
   Includes bibliographical references and index.
   ISBN 0-7373-0361-1 (alk. paper)
      1. Gastrointestinal system—Diseases. 2. Nutrition—Health aspects. I. Title.
  RC806 .R525 2001
  616.3'3—dc21

                                               2001042234

Contemporary Books

A Division of The **McGraw·Hill** Companies

1 2 3 4 5 6 7 8 9 10   DOC/DOC   1 10 9 8 7 6 5 4 3 2

ISBN 0-7373-0361-1

This book was typeset in Lydian and Minion by Robert S. Tinnon Design
Printed and bound by R. R. Donnelley—Crawfordsville
Cover design by Mike Stromberg/The Great American Art Co.
Interior design by Robert S. Tinnon

McGraw-Hill books are available at special quantity discounts to use as
premiums and sales promotions, or for use in corporate training programs.
For more information, please write to the Director of Special Sales, Professional
Publishing, McGraw-Hill, Two Penn Plaza, New York, NY 10121-2298.
Or contact your local bookstore.

This book is printed on acid-free paper.

To John, who makes beautiful music and can build or
fix anything, a true Renaissance man and
a St. Francis of Assisi for the new millennium; and
to the memory of his mother, Mary Catherine Reinhard,
a warm and giving person who taught
two generations about health and nutrition.

To Gea DeRubeis-Pacifico (a piece of gum really
does help you digest, which makes me wonder how many
other things you said were really true!), and to Guy Pacifico,
gravy train conductor and financial wizard,
whose generosity has made possible Faye and
Brendan's love of Barisciano and everything
Italian, as has their Grandma Pacifico's
exquisite culinary talent.

Contents

■ . . . . . . ■

Acknowledgments

■ · · · · · · ■

Thanks to Shelley Baker, R.D., and Lynn Kuligowski, R.D., Wayne State University dietetics graduates, two of the smartest and nicest people I know, for help with research. Many thanks to a wonderful aspiring artist, Rosanna Kisovic, for her great drawings. Thanks also to Dr. Leora Shelef who once gave me a food science book when I really needed one; to Joyce Mooty, M.A., M.Ed., R.D., an incredible dietitian and educator who taught me all about bezoars; and to Dr. David Klurfeld, the doctor who is always in and who continues to inspire young scientific minds as well as the rest of us!

Introduction

■ · · · · · · ■

It was 2:30 A.M. I was flipping pages in yet another oversized textbook and sipping my now-cold tea. I was determined to develop an intriguing and meaningful lecture for the university job I had started one week before: teaching medical school hopefuls and future dietitians about nutrition and health. For that first lecture, I planned to teach them all there was to know about diseases of the gastrointestinal (GI) tract. Then my sleep-starved eyes latched on to a quotation from gastroenterologist K. B. Taylor, a quotation I'd eventually print on an overhead slide and show for the next ten years in the same class.

> Many such diets suggest more the physician treating himself rather than the patient, and the results were not always harmless.[1]

The quote sounded a familiar chord. I'd talked to countless patients who had given up many of their favorite foods, some of which were quite nutritious, because the foods turned up on the "not allowed" side of a printed diet sheet for a variety of GI ills. The problem was that the latest research showed that many of these GI diets rarely had benefit. For instance, Taylor cited the case of a sixty-year-old woman who developed scurvy (vitamin C deficiency); her physician had advised her twenty years earlier to eliminate all fruits and vegetables from her diet to treat indigestion. Her doctor died before rescinding his advice.

Although that example is rather dramatic, it highlights potential problems with the "one-size-fits-all" approach of traditional diets used to treat GI disorders. Whenever foods, and especially whole groups of foods, are eliminated from a diet, so are the nutrients that those foods contain. Another problem, no less important, is that rigid diets often impose needless dietary hardship or monotony, a direct violation of the first dietary guideline for Americans: "Eat a variety of foods."

If studies have shown that a particular diet improves the GI problem, its benefits probably outweigh its risks, but if there is no proof of a diet's effectiveness, all you have is risk. Would you take a pill, one with unpleasant and maybe adverse side effects, if the drug company hadn't proved that the pill works? Here are four questions to ask about any GI diet you might be considering or are already following for more than a few weeks.

1. Is the diet nutritionally adequate?
2. Is the diet acceptable to you?
3. Have scientists studied the diet and shown its potential value in treating disease?
4. Are there any undesirable side effects that can occur due to following the diet?

Unfortunately, many GI diets popular in recent years weren't meeting two, let alone all four, criteria. A GI diet should always be tailored to each individual to account for that person's specific intolerances. Even if a particular food hasn't been shown to affect a GI disorder, it may cause problems for one person and not another with the same disease. Regardless of whether the person actually has a physical intolerance to the food, a belief that the food will cause problems often ensures that it will.

When you consider the importance of the GI tract's key roles in maintaining life and health, it's easy to see how profoundly GI diseases can affect a person's nutritional health and ultimately his or her overall health. The GI tract's main functions are to ingest and digest food so that the nutrients it contains can be absorbed into the system and, once that's done, to get rid of whatever remains that wasn't needed by the body. When something goes wrong with the GI system, it doesn't take long before nutritional health suffers. A person in poor nutritional health can't support a healthy immune system; therefore, that person is more likely to succumb to infection and illness than is a healthy person.

Another quote I give to my students as we begin the study of GI diseases comes from Shakespeare's *Macbeth*. It shows how time-honored and universal is the understanding that a properly functioning GI system is crucial for good health: "Good digestions wait on appetite and health on both."

This book starts with an overview of the GI tract: how it works and the kinds of problems that can arise. The chapters that follow focus on the diseases of the upper GI tract and the lower GI tract. Along the way comes a look at new research into the causes and treatments of GI diseases, with special emphasis on potentially helpful nutrition regimens.

PART I

Overview of Gastrointestinal Disorders

■ · · · · · · ■

" It was a searing pain and feeling of tightness that started in my chest and spread out all over my upper body." It sounded like a potential heart attack, which made this friendly middle-aged woman's admitting diagnosis of possible myocardial infarction quite logical. My routine nutrition screening questions had quickly changed to pointed questions on her recent weight loss. "Now they say I didn't have a heart attack after all; the antibiotics I was taking made an ulcer in my throat," the woman told me. An ulcer would explain her poor appetite, which in turn caused severe weight loss over the past month or so. Unfortunately, for the next few days and maybe longer, her diet would be a clear liquid regimen.

This woman's situation illustrates how something as everyday as a common antibiotic can affect the GI tract and wreak havoc on nutritional status and health. Her pain was caused by a sphincter separating the esophagus from the stomach staying closed when it should have opened, leaving the antibiotic in contact with the delicate tissue of the esophagus.

The complexity of the simple act of swallowing, or the deceptively basic opening and closing of a sphincter, gives rise to the numerous GI problems for which patients see their doctors. *Dyspepsia*, the medical term for indigestion, is the reason for more than 50 percent of all visits to internists every year. Some cases will have easy fixes, such as eliminating a certain food or taking a medication, whereas the vast majority will go undiagnosed or untreated. Yet other GI problems will be identified as chronic conditions that will dramatically change a patient's life forever.

This part starts with a look at all the interconnecting parts of the GI tract, their functions, and the problems that can affect each one.

CHAPTER I

How It Works
(When It Does Work)

■　·　·　·　·　·　·　■

Another name for the GI tract, the *gut*, generally gets a few laughs from my students, although I tell them that even the gut experts, gastroenterologists, use this term. Its name may be funny, but its jobs are serious: ingest, digest, absorb, and excrete food components. Several organs and tissues are involved in these processes. The GI tract begins with the mouth and ends with the anus, and in between, organs such as the liver, gallbladder, and pancreas get in on the action (see Figure 1.1 and Table 1.1). To want to ingest food, a person must experience hunger or appetite, both of which start in the brain. Therefore, how a person is feeling emotionally can upset the whole process.

With so many organs involved, a problem in any one can have a profound effect on the process and therefore on nutritional status and health. If the entire length of only the small intestine were laid out and slit open from end to end, the surface area would cover approximately one quarter of a football field. It is therefore easy for some type of damage to occur in some part of the gut, because so much of it is exposed to mechanical, thermal, chemical, and microbial damage after a lifetime of eating every four hours or so.

This chapter takes a tour of the GI tract, starting with chewing food in the mouth to the final steps of absorbing nutrients and excreting the parts of the food that are not used.

THE MOUTH

The average American probably spends three and a quarter years chewing food. That amazing amount of time is time well spent. Many of the most common GI problems often have their start in this "mini-garbage disposal." Take gas, for instance: inadequate chewing can cause this common GI condition. Indigestion, another typical reason for people to head to the doctor's office, can also develop from eating too

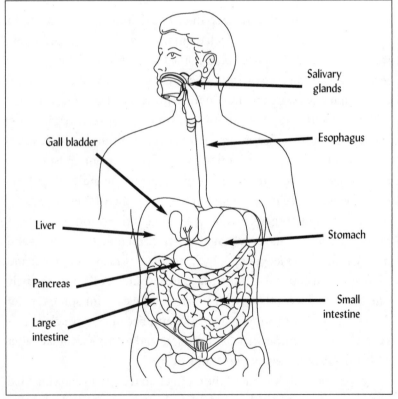

Figure 1.1 The Digestive System

quickly. Most Americans do eat too quickly, and too often they eat fast foods. Over the years, Americans have taken to eating in their cars and at their work desks. Between dodging other vehicles on the freeway and talking to the boss between gulps of a bologna sandwich, it's easy to see that we all need to slow it down.

Table 1.1 Overview of the Digestive System

Organ/Tissue	What It Secretes	What It Does
Salivary glands	Saliva; salivary amylase	Liquefies food, begins digestion of starch
Stomach	Gastric juice; enzymes; acid	Begins digestion of protein, converts minerals for absorption
	Intrinsic factor	Allows for vitamin B_{12} absorption
	Mucus	Protects stomach cells
Small intestine	Intestinal juice; enzymes	Digests carbohydrate, protein
	Mucus	Protects intestinal cells
	Hormones	Regulate digestion
Pancreas	Pancreatic juice; bicarbonate	Reduces acidity, activates enzymes
	Enzymes	Digest carbohydrate, protein, fat
Gallbladder	Bile[a]	Emulsifies fat so that it can be digested

[a]Bile is made by the liver and stored and ejected by the gallbladder.

Slowing down the chewing process itself has rewards. Taking longer to eat a meal gives your stomach a chance to realize that it's full. Feeling full is usually the signal for most people to stop eating, so weight loss and management may be an easier task. Other payoffs may be more important, such as a decreased likelihood of choking. To a young, healthy person, this payoff may not seem like much, but it could save the life of an older person. As we age, the swallowing mechanism is not as strong as it is in our youth, and swallowing problems have become increasingly prevalent as the U. S. population has aged. When a person has difficulty swallowing, the risk for choking increases significantly.

To chew food properly, the teeth and gums need to be in top shape. A common problem for older people with dentures is that over time, changes in the gums can cause dentures to not fit properly. When dentures don't fit, eating becomes difficult and even painful. Many conditions aside from poor dental health can also affect the ability to chew food properly. Some common problems include mouth or gum surgery, reduced saliva flow, and mouth sores or ulcers that make it painful to eat. Many diseases can cause these last two conditions, as can a variety of drugs. Radiation therapy also causes mouth ulcers.

THE ESOPHAGUS

Everyone marvels at the old movie reels showing the red-caped circus performer swallowing blazing yard-long torches, but even the mundane act of swallowing morning eggs and toast should impress us. As with most of the hidden intricacies of the wonderful machine called the human body, the amazing act of swallowing is only noticed when something goes wrong, such as a sore throat. Unlike many life-sustaining processes that take place without a person's will or even awareness, the involuntary processes, the first step in swallowing is voluntary.

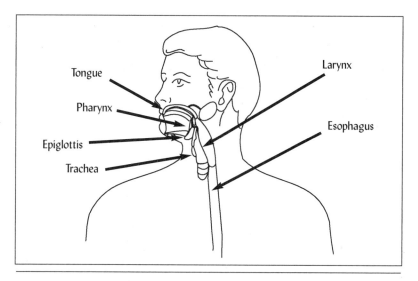

Figure 1.2 The structures involved in the swallowing process

This first voluntary step in swallowing is part of a complicated three-stage process, and once it begins, reflexes take over to finish the act (see Figure 1.2). Each stage takes its name from the structure that dominates the step: oral, pharyngeal, and esophageal. The act takes five to ten seconds from start to finish. The first stage is the oral phase: a person puts food in the mouth, then mixes it with saliva and chews, which help to predigest the food and make it easier to swallow. The tongue plays a role in this phase by forming the chewed food into a round lump called a *bolus* and pushing it toward the back of the mouth by slowly squeezing the bolus back up against the hard and soft palates.

The next step is the pharyngeal phase, which starts when the bolus reaches the faucial arches. In this phase, quick ministeps need to occur: the soft palate rises to shut the opening of the pharynx; the pharynx rises and the vocal cords move toward the middle to close the airway, temporarily preventing breathing; and the pharynx begins to tighten and a connecting sphincter relaxes, letting food slip into the esophagus. At that point, the person is able to breathe again. In the final, involuntary phase, the esophageal, the muscles of the esophagus, move the bolus into the stomach by peristaltic waves, with the help of gravity. Numerous problems, all classed under *dysphagia*, can arise in each step, and can lead to serious complications.

THE STOMACH

The big show starts in the stomach. In this dynamic acid pit, which also serves as a holding tank, the real work of breaking down food and getting it into small enough components that the body can use begins. Shaped like half a valentine heart, the stomach is connected at the top to the esophagus and at its lower end to the small intestine (see Figure 1.3). The stomach in some ways is a checkpoint for the digestion and absorption process. The job of the esophagus is to conduct the swallowed food into the stomach. The small intestine fine-tunes digestion to allow nutrients to be absorbed across its surface. The stomach keeps the two in sync with various hormones and nerves that allow the GI tract to act in harmony.

A quick look at the anatomy of the stomach shows this organ's elegant and task-specific design. The stomach is divided into three parts: fundus, body, and pylorus. The fundus is the upper portion that arches upward away from the opening to the esophagus. That opening to the esophagus is guarded by a circular band of muscle fibers—called the *lower esophageal*, or *cardiac, sphincter* (LES)—that can open and close as needed. This little sphincter closes to keep the contents of the stomach in the stomach and opens to allow food to pass from the esophagus into the stomach.

The body of the stomach is between the fundus and the lower portion, the pylorus. Another sphincter, the pyloric, guards the opening between the stomach and the small intestine. The failure of these sphincters to open and close at the right time is the cause of many GI symptoms and disorders.

The stomach, and for that matter the entire GI tract, consists of layers of muscle, some going in different directions. This muscle layering allows the gut to move in the rhythmic manner of a snake swallowing its prey. In much the same way, peristalsis moves the food from the esophagus to the stomach in regular waves. This peristaltic movement also physically grinds the food to a pastelike consistency. Peristalsis keeps the paste moving along in the small intestine so that nutrients can be absorbed. Finally, this rhythmic movement pushes the waste product through the colon so that it can be eliminated.

Back in the stomach, glands and specialized cells begin digestion and prepare the food for final digestion in the small intestine. Epithelial cells form the surface layer of the mucous membrane, or *mucosa*,

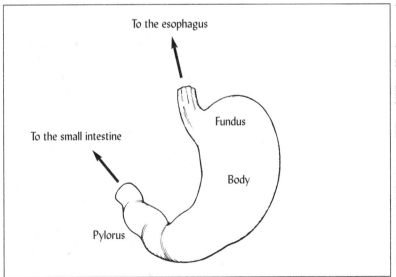

Figure 1.3 The Human Stomach

that lines the inside of the stomach. The mucosa protects the deeper layers of stomach tissue by secreting thick mucus. Only a few compounds, such as water and salts, can cross the membrane. This design continues through the gut: in the stomach it's called *gastric mucosa,* and in the small intestine, it's called *intestinal mucosa.*

Another type of cell, parietal cells located in the fundus, secretes hydrochloric acid and a compound known as the intrinsic factor. Acid breaks apart the protein in food. Proteins are coiled into different shapes, much like a Slinky. For enzymes to get at connecting points, or bonds, between atoms of the protein, the protein has to be uncoiled in a process called *denaturation.* An everyday example of protein denaturation is adding vinegar or lemon juice, both quite acidic, to a protein-containing food such as milk. The resulting clotting is the milk protein being denatured. Acid also activates enzymes that assist in breaking down protein and changes some nutrients into a form that will be better absorbed in the small intestine. The intrinsic factor is necessary for the absorption of vitamin B_{12} in the last portion of the small intestine. Without this vital compound, a person would not be able to absorb this important vitamin and would need regular injections of B_{12}. People who have had major gastric surgery, with much or all of the stomach removed, need such injections.

Stomach glands in the mucosa secrete gastric juice, which contains everything the stomach needs to begin digestion, such as enzymes, more acid, and protective mucus. Chief cells secrete digestive enzymes that start to break down protein and, to a lesser extent, fat from food. Most of the digestion, however, takes place in the small intestine. The real work of the stomach is to grind the food to a paste consistency, which happens in the antrum of the stomach. When the stomach has some of the food in this form, called *chyme,* it begins a two-way communication with the small intestine whereby small amounts of chyme will proceed to enter the small intestine at a controlled rate.

The stomach and the small intestine talk to each other by a set of nerve and hormone connections. This critical communication ensures that the stomach empties at a pace that works for both the stomach and the intestine. For example, if food empties from the stomach too quickly, the small intestine doesn't have enough time to neutralize the acidity. This high acidity could damage the intestinal membrane because it is not protected from acid like the stomach is. In addition, the quick emptying doesn't give the stomach time to break down the food mechanically to the paste consistency. The result of quick emptying would be a load of large food particles into the small intestine and movement of fluid from surrounding tissue into the lumen of the intestine, causing bloating, pain, and diarrhea. Another consequence of rapid stomach emptying is that the small intestine doesn't have enough time to digest the food and absorb the nutrients it contains, which could lead to malnutrition.

THE SMALL INTESTINE

At 21 feet long and with the daunting responsibility of digesting and absorbing everything a person eats and drinks, there is nothing small about this organ. Its 1-inch diameter makes it small in comparison to the diameter of the large intestine, which is more than double, averaging 2½ inches. The first 10 inches of the small intestine is the duodenum, the next 8 feet is the jejunem, and the last 12 feet is the ileum (see Figure 1.4).

The tissue of the small intestine is similar to the rest of the GI tract in that layers of muscles enable the important peristaltic movement responsible for conducting food through the gut. If peristalsis occurs too quickly, *hypermotility* (excessive movement of the muscles of the GI tract), diarrhea, and even malnutrition can result. The opposite scenario, poor motility or movement, causes abdominal problems and constipation.

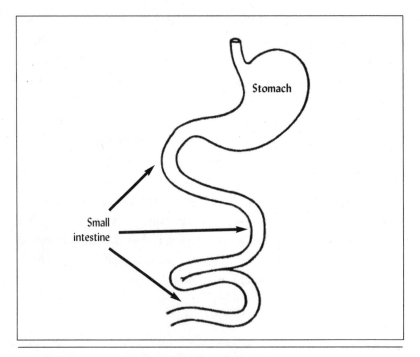

Figure 1.4 The Small Intestine

The folds in the interior of the small intestine greatly increase its surface area, allowing more nutrients to be absorbed from foods. Intestinal mucosal cells, the specialized cells that line the organ, release enzymes to first break down nutrients; then the nutrients can enter the cells. Once inside the cell, nutrients are transported across from the surface to the basement membrane, which is adjacent to tiny blood vessels called *capillaries*, in a process known as *absorption*. After entering the capillary, a nutrient is free to travel through the bloodstream and make its way to where it is needed, very often preceded by a stop in the liver for special processing or packaging.

The three different sections of the small intestine each have their own responsibilities regarding the absorption of specific nutrients (see Figure 1.5). In addition to secreting digestive enzymes, the duodenum

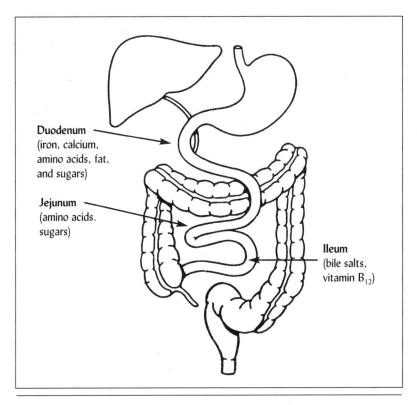

Figure 1.5 Nutrient Absorption Sites in the Small Intestine

absorbs vitamin A, thiamin, iron, calcium, amino acids, glycerol and fatty acids, and sugars. It is in the duodenum that the common bile duct makes its entry. This duct brings the digestive secretions of the gallbladder and the pancreas into the small intestine, where all the action is. These digestive helpers assist in the breakdown of fat, carbohydrate, and protein. The gallbladder secretes bile, a chemical that emulsifies fat so that digestive enzymes can break it down, whereas the liver makes bile.

The pancreas secretes digestive enzymes and bicarbonate, which neutralizes the acidity of the chyme. Bicarbonate is important for two reasons. First, the duodenum is not specially equipped to handle acid as is the stomach and could become physically damaged and form ulcers. Second, the enzymes of the small intestine are only active at a neutral pH (acid) level. The next stop is the jejunem, where more amino acids and sugars are absorbed, and the final stop is the ileum, where vitamin B_{12} and bile are absorbed. Diseases that strike specific areas of the small intestine can cause a deficiency of whichever nutrient should have been digested and absorbed in that location.

Although the liver receives most of the absorbed nutrients, some nutrients must rely on dietary fat for absorption. After it has been split into smaller components that can enter the intestinal cell, dietary fat and fat-soluble nutrients such as vitamins A, D, E, and K travel through a special transport system called the *lymphatics*. Once all the nutrients have been absorbed from the food, what's left is waste, which needs to be eliminated. Waste includes any food components that couldn't be digested, such as various types of fiber. The waste exits the small intestine and enters the large intestine for the last leg of the journey.

THE LARGE INTESTINE

In some ways, the large intestine has an easy job. By the time what's left of the food mass moves to this organ, digestion has taken place and all the important nutrients have been absorbed. The large intestine reabsorbs some water, gases, and electrolytes (minerals such as sodium and potassium), but its main function is to excrete the waste.

The large intestine is a 6-foot tube about the diameter of a vacuum cleaner hose, with several different sections. The first segment, about the first 3 inches, is the cecum, which is followed by four segments of colon: ascending, transverse, descending, and sigmoid colons (see Figure 1.6). The last 7 inches is the rectum leading to the anus, which is guarded by two sphincter muscles. It takes about twenty-four hours

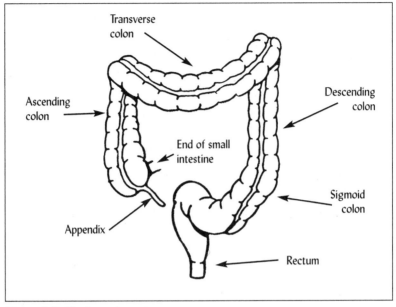

Figure 1.6 The Large Intestine

for food residue to reach the colon and up to seventy-two hours for consumed food to be excreted in a process called *defecation*. Many factors influence the time it takes from ingestion of food to excretion, which is known as transit time, including diet composition, water intake, and physical activity. A variety of prescription medications can also affect transit time, causing either diarrhea or constipation.

As with the small intestine, many diseases of the large intestine tend to strike specific areas of the organ. Fortunately, because the large intestine isn't involved in nutrient digestion and absorption, a person can expect to have a normal life span even if the entire organ must be removed as a result of disease. In the past, the large intestine was thought to be passive, but recent research has pointed to the health importance of processes that take place only here. In contrast to the small intestine, the healthy colon is inhabited by friendly bacteria.

These little bugs help keep a person healthy in several ways, the most basic of which is by keeping down populations of bad bacteria that cause disease. In addition, the friendly bacteria possess digestive enzymes that the human body does not. Thus, as food components that the body cannot digest, such as fiber, enter the large intestine, the bugs break down these components. Although the amount of nutrients released are probably minimal (aside from vitamin K, a necessary vitamin that the body receives only in this way), the by-products have turned out to be intriguing compounds: short-chain fatty acids. Scientists studying these fatty acids speculate that they help keep the colon moving briskly, feed the organ's surface cells, and may reduce the risk for cancer.

CHAPTER 2

What Goes Wrong and How Diet Can Help

■ · · · · · · ■

After what we've just learned about the complexity of a seemingly simple act—nourishing our bodies—it's easy to see how minor glitches can occur. A functional problem in any organ or specialized tissue involved in digestion and absorption will throw a wrench into the entire process. In addition, the surface of the GI tract is continually exposed to millions of potentially toxic agents from the foods we eat. The more years we've been digesting and absorbing, the more likely problems will occur. Of course, young people can be affected as well.

In general, most intestinal problems are functional; in other words, the tissues are not functioning as they should. These problems involve motility, absorption, or secretion. Motility problems can involve inadequate mixing of food in the GI tract or too much or too little propulsion of the waste products. Problems with absorption in the stomach, small intestine, or colon can produce symptoms ranging from gassiness to chronic diarrhea and malnutrition. Any compound the GI tract releases during normal digestion and absorption—such as enzymes, hormones, mucus, electrolytes, and water—constitutes a secretion. Of course, some problems are structural in origin, such as a tumor in the stomach. Eventually, however, a structural problem will affect function.

The overriding principle in diet therapy for gastrointestinal disease is that the diet needs to be highly individualized. Not only can a specific disease evolve somewhat differently in different people, but because much of the intestinal tract's work is under the control of nerve impulses and hormones, both of which are intricately linked with a person's psyche and state of mind, the placebo effect can play a part. Also key in the dietary approach to GI disease is that, with few exceptions, diet therapy cannot cure a disease. Changes in diet can, however, help alleviate symptoms and maintain nutritional health.

These foundational principles translate into the two major dietary treatment objectives applicable to all GI diseases: control GI symptoms and maintain good nutritional status. These objectives may not sound like much, but failure to achieve them not only adversely affects quality of life but may end it prematurely. As we look at the many diseases of the upper and lower GI tract and at dietary approaches, remember to apply the following criteria to any regimen: the diet must be nutritionally adequate, acceptable to the patient, have scientific evidence for its effectiveness, and not present any undesirable side effects.

THE MOST BASIC GI DIET:
CHANGING TEXTURE AND CONSISTENCY

Although specific GI diseases involve a dietary regimen, very often the diet will need to be changed for reasons that are mechanical in nature. For example, starting at the beginning of the GI tract, conditions such as mouth sores, major dental problems, or surgery make it difficult for a person to chew and swallow food adequately. In those cases, food must be in a form that will require minimal or no chewing action to make it the proper consistency for the esophagus and stomach. At other times, because of disease or injury affecting that segment, it may be necessary to bypass the first segments of the intestine and put nutrients into the next GI segment through a tube. Finally, and more serious, is the need to bypass the GI tract altogether and put nutrients directly into the bloodstream.

Mechanical Soft and Pureed Diets

A chewing or swallowing problem requires a change in the diet's texture and consistency. The mechanical diet (also called a dental soft, or edentulous, diet) excludes foods that are typically difficult to chew or swallow. It can consist merely of processing hard-to-chew foods, such as grinding tough meats. This minor change should be taken seriously because it can affect a person's appetite. Often, the excluded foods may be a person's favorites, or the processing—usually chopping, blending, overcooking, or adding extra liquid—can make foods unappealing. Therefore, a dietitian should work closely with the patient and caregivers to prevent a drop in food intake and an unintentional weight loss.

The mechanical soft diet can be taken a step further, a big step, with the pureed diet. In this diet, foods are strained and blended to a thickened, almost liquid, state. In the past, some hospitals merely opened jars of baby food and poured the contents into separate bowls, presenting the hapless patient with a tray of three or four small white dishes containing glops of materials rumored to be roast beef, sweet potatoes, and green beans. Even more mind-boggling was the food service technique in which all the whole foods on the menu for a meal were dumped into a giant stainless steel blender, poured into one large styrofoam cup, and placed, with a long straw, before the patient! It's easy to see how any food-loving person would decide that eating was not worth it. Today, advances in food technology have made it possible to serve pureed foods, such as lasagna and peanut butter and jelly sandwiches, that actually look like their unpureed counterparts. Unfortunately, these ready-to-use items are expensive. An alternative is to add special commercial thickeners to pureed food, which gives the food better form and makes it more appetizing.

Enteral and Parenteral Nutrition

Enteral nutrition uses the GI tract to introduce nutrients, whereas parenteral nutrition bypasses the GI tract and places nutrients directly into the blood. Modern enteral and parenteral nutrition, often collectively called *nutrition support,* has its roots in NASA's efforts in the 1950s to make space travel nutritionally safe. Historians say that the practice actually goes back to the ancient Egyptians and Greeks. Physicians fed President James Garfield this way after he was shot in 1881.

It's always preferable to use the GI tract rather than the bloodstream for feeding when possible. First, fewer complications, such as infection, a lung puncture, or blood vessel collapse, are likely. Second, enteral nutrition is more like normal feeding, because the GI tract is used. When the GI tract is bypassed entirely, the intestinal mucosal cells atrophy, or lose their integrity over time. When deciding which form of nutrition support to use, the traditional maxim is, "If the gut works, use it, and if it works a little, use it a little."

Enteral Nutrition Once the physician decides to use enteral nutrition, several more decisions still need to be made. At this time, it is advisable to team up with a dietitian. Two basic decisions are where the tube will enter the GI tract (the entry point) and in what part of the GI tract it will deliver the feeding (the delivery point). Several factors influence these decisions, including the area of the GI tract that needs to be bypassed; the person's risk for *aspiration,* or the taking of foreign matter into the lungs when breathing; and the length of time the person will need the tube feeding. The entry points include the nose, esophagus, stomach, duodenum, and jejunem; all except the nose require a surgical incision. Because the nasal passages are sensitive and cannot withstand tube feeding for very long, the typical limit for nose feeding is about two weeks. If the tube feeding needs to go on longer, another entry point will be needed.

The decision about the tube feeding delivery point is based on risk for aspiration and the need to bypass a segment of the GI tract. The risk for aspiration is greatly reduced when the stomach is bypassed. If, however, aspiration risk is low and the stomach is working, feeding in the stomach is better because it simulates the natural process more closely.

Most people who need tube feedings only need them for a short time, usually while recovering from an illness in the hospital. Some people, however, will continue tube feedings in their homes, which requires close consultation with a dietitian.

Tube feedings, called *formulas,* are highly specialized, often disease-specific, products. Most provide all the essential nutrients in a day's supply, although some nutrients may be higher or lower, depending on the dietary regimen imposed by the patient's special needs. Although enteral nutrition poses fewer risks than parenteral, complications can arise. A common problem is abdominal distress, notably distension and diarrhea. If the diarrhea is persistent, caregivers need to reduce the rate at which the formula is infused. Often, the GI tract gets used to the feeding, and the rate can soon be increased.

Parenteral Nutrition When a person's GI tract isn't functioning at all, the only way to get that person the nutrition needed is to insert it into a blood vessel, via a needle attached to a catheter. The physician needs to decide into which vessel to insert the needle and what the specific contents of the nutritional solution should be. The main factor guiding this decision is the length of time the person will need parenteral nutrition. If short term, about two weeks, a peripheral blood vessel, in an arm or leg, will be used; this method is called *peripheral* *parenteral nutrition.* Infusing the nutrient solution into peripheral vessels for more than two weeks can cause the vessels to collapse. If parenteral nutrition will be longer than two weeks, only a central vein, a large-diameter vessel near the heart, can be used. This type of parenteral nutrition, called *central parenteral* or *total parenteral nutrition,* is more risky compared to peripheral parenteral for two reasons. First is the possibility of accidentally puncturing a lung or the heart. Second, inserting a catheter so close to the heart makes infection—one that would quickly spread throughout the body—more likely. A person with a GI disease or injury requiring removal of more than 75 percent of the small intestine will need total parenteral nutrition for the rest of his or her life, and in this regard, this method has been a lifesaver. Unfortunately, long-term complications such as infections, fatty liver, and abnormal blood values for various constituents can arise.

A WORD ABOUT RESEARCH STUDIES

Nutrition researchers like to say that their field of study is a young science. Although this science has an illustrious and intriguing history, most of the major research advances have occurred relatively recently, an important point to remember in any study of GI diseases. An update on recent research with discussions of specific diseases follows in Parts II and III. Figure 2.1 gives some guidelines for evaluating research results.

For study results to be truly valid, other researchers have to repeat the same experiment and come to the same conclusions. If the results of a study can be reproduced in similar studies, the conclusions are considered reliable.

Scientists can use one of four basic types of studies to prove a hypothesis, and each type has its pros and cons (see Table 2.1). The type of study most people know about is the laboratory study, which uses test tubes (in vitro) or animals and which provides details on how

- Laboratory studies (tissue cultures, animals) are not necessarily applicable to humans; they can only point the way for human studies.
- Epidemiologic studies show statistical associations that may or may not indicate cause and effect. They also point the way for human trials.
- Human trials are the most powerful studies, but the results need to be repeated to be considered valid and for the treatment to be safe and effective.
- The number of subjects in a human study is important; the larger the study group, the more likely the results are valid.
- In human studies, results are more likely to be valid when the subjects were similar (age, gender, etc.); then, however, the results may not apply to people who are different from the subjects.

Figure 2.1 Tips for Evaluating Research Results

a specific effect works. For example, in an in vitro lab study of glutamine, an amino acid that may be helpful in some types of GI disease, scientists add glutamine to cultured tissue samples in a lab dish and watch what happens. In an animal study, researchers inject glutamine into a rat.

In an epidemiological study, scientists study disease in a specific population. For example, a study could compare the rate of ulcerative colitis among Americans in the South with different levels of glutamine in their diets. The ultimate study would be a clinical trial testing glutamine in a group of people with ulcerative colitis and comparing them with a similar number of people with the disease who don't get the treatment.

The obvious shortcoming in in vitro lab studies using only cells is that the cells in the dish may not react the same way as those in a living person's small intestine. One benefit of animal studies is that the animals can be dissected later and then studied for many details on

Table 2.1 Types of Research Studies

Study Type	What Is It?	Pro	Con
Laboratory	Animal studies	Similarity of subjects	An animal is not a person, so results cannot be applied
		Can use numerous subjects	
		Can dissect subjects to learn more	
		Usually of short duration (based on life span of animal)	
	In vitro doesn't use a living organism; uses tissues	Inexpensive	Less validity because not in a living or chemical organism
		Short-duration experiment	
Case study	Follows the clinical course of one person	Human study; more valid than animal or in vitro	Less validity because only one person observed
Epidemiologic	Compares populations of people with regard to some aspect of diet	Large numbers, more valid	Cannot show disease incidence and cause and effect; only statistical correlation

Continued

Table 2.1 *Continued*

Study Type	What Is It?	Pro	Con
Intervention/ clinical trial	Human study comparing the effects of a treatment to no treatment or a different treatment	Good validity, applicability to other people	Very expensive

Note: Even the best results of any type of study must be replicated by other studies before they can be considered valid.

glutamine's effects. An animal's intestine may not respond the same way a person's intestine might, however, so other scientists will have to do another study with humans. Therein lies the main usefulness of the lab study: it points researchers in the right direction. The epidemiological study can't prove conclusively that people with higher intakes of glutamine are protected against the disease, but it can establish statistical association, giving researchers a clue as to whether the question is worth pursuing with expensive and long clinical trials.

Remember that all studies have their limitations, and even the best human trials need to be repeated and show the same results before physicians can use the approach safely and effectively.

PART II

Diseases of the
Upper Gastrointestinal Tract

■ · · · · · · ■

I watched fascinated as my spry uncle painstakingly peeled the soft peach. I had never seen anyone peel this fruit, and as the peel came away in one long, spiral strip, drops of juice ran down his hands. When I asked my mother why he had peeled the peach, she told me that the peach skin could hurt his ulcers. I was only six years old at the time, but similar stories cropped up decades later when I was counseling patients with upper GI problems such as ulcers. Research has since shown that many of these strict food practices had no basis in fact. For example, today my uncle's ulcer would be treated with antibiotics and most probably never bother him again. On the flip side, the connection between our heads and our stomachs cannot be denied. Scientists call an improvement in a condition that cannot be specifically traced to treatment the *placebo effect.*

So what's the problem with believing that the peel on a fuzzy peach will hurt your ulcer? It is probably not much of a problem for some people, but others won't take the time to peel the peach and will instead opt not to eat it. The more limited a person's diet becomes—and very often limited in highly nutritious fruits and vegetables—the more likely a deficiency is to crop up. In the case of the fuzzy peel, there's a healthy supply of vitamins directly under the skin of any piece of fruit. Getting the most nutrients out of food should be everyone's nutrition and health goal.

CHAPTER 3

Diseases of the Esophagus

■ · · · · · · ■

DYSPHAGIA

Simply stated, dysphagia is difficulty in swallowing. The reasons for the difficulty are diverse (see Figure 3.1), and dysphagia's most common victims are the elderly. As more Americans join the ranks of the elderly, the number of people affected by dysphagia is sure to increase. Some of the causes are the aging process, stroke, physical disabilities, and multiple sclerosis or any disease affecting the nervous system. In addition, many people who have had a temporary nasogastric tube (i.e., were fed through the nose) for a significant length of time may experience short-term dysphagia. In some ways, it's hard to imagine that swallowing, a simple act most people don't ever think about, can cause such serious problems. The most serious one is that food may enter the trachea, causing the person to choke. Another problem is when the choking reflex is affected by dysphagia, so that food enters the trachea and the lungs, where bacteria multiply and cause pneumonia. This situation is called *silent aspiration*.

- Aging
- AIDS
- Alzheimer's disease
- Brain tumor, head or neck cancer, head injury
- Developmental disabilities
- Guillain-Barré syndrome
- Lou Gehrig's disease (amyotrophic lateral sclerosis)
- Multiple sclerosis
- Myasthenia gravis
- Parkinson's disease
- Polio
- Reflux esophagitis
- Stroke

Figure 3.1 Causes of Dysphagia

Symptoms and Diagnosis

It's easy to miss the signs of dysphagia, particularly in the elderly. Health professionals and caregivers are usually the first to notice a swallowing problem in elderly patients under their care. Common indirect symptoms include poor food intake and weight loss and frequent diagnosis of pneumonia. More obvious symptoms are painful swallowing, drooling, complaints that food is sticking in the throat, excessive swallowing, and pocketing food between the teeth and cheek. A caregiver may notice that a person with dysphagia clears his or her throat excessively or coughs while eating.

Several tests can help diagnose or determine the severity of swallowing problems (see Figure 3.2). By the use of a specialized scope called

Esophagogastroduodenoscopy (upper GI endoscopy, gastroscopy, EGD [esophagus, stomach, and duodenum]): Technicians insert a long, flexible tube (endoscope) equipped with a fiber-optic–lighted scope into the patient's mouth to allow health care professionals to see inside various organs (the lumen) of the digestive tract. The endoscope can have up to three channels to allow for viewing, suffusion of air or aspiration (removal) of fluid, and biopsy of tissue. It can reach into the duodenum (first part of the small intestine). In addition to diagnosing problems, it can be used to treat conditions such as GI bleeding.

Esophageal function studies: After fasting, the patient swallows up to three tubes equipped with pressure-detecting devices. The tubes pass into the stomach, and as they do so, pressure in the esophagus is recorded. The tubes are slowly pulled back into the esophagus, providing a pressure reading for the LES sphincter. The patient swallows, which shows the peristaltic wave pattern. Next, acid is infused into the stomach through one of the tubes, which provides information on whether acid is coming back up (refluxing) from the stomach into the esophagus and on the patient's ability to clear acid from the esophagus.

Barium swallow (esophagogram): After fasting for eight hours, the patient drinks a milkshake type of beverage containing barium (a radiographic material that allows the esophagus to be visualized; also called a *contrast agent*). The technician asks the patient to roll into different positions so that the entire esophagus is visible. The health care professional can watch the barium flow through the esophagus by immediately projecting the image on a fluorescent screen; images can be captured on X-ray film. The results enable the health care team to distinguish among a neurologic cause, a problem with the sphincter, the presence of tumors, inflammation, and other conditions, which makes treatment more specific and effective.

Videofluoroscopy swallowing examination: The patient swallows food items to which barium has been added, and the process is videotaped. Later, health care professionals can watch the entire swallowing process to determine what and where the problem is.

Figure 3.2 Swallowing Evaluation Tests

an *endoscope*, which includes a pressure-detecting device, and X rays, physicians can see the peristaltic waves of the esophagus, measure the pressure in the sphincter, and find out if acid is coming up from the stomach into the esophagus, a condition called *reflux*. If a hospitalized patient is suspected of having swallowing problems, a speech pathologist will conduct a swallowing evaluation at the bedside. This evaluation consists of providing the patient with several different food items and observing his or her reaction to determine the food texture and consistency that may present problems. In addition to diagnosing dysphagia, the swallowing evaluation is used by the speech pathologist when working with the dietitian to plan a proper diet.

Research Update on Dysphagia

Researchers at Wayne State University in Detroit studied the therapeutic effects of botulinum toxin (Botox) in patients with dysphagia. This toxin is the same agent that causes botulism, a potentially deadly disease. The study included five patients whose dysphagia was caused by muscle spasm and/or hypertonicity (abnormally high muscle strength or tone). Researchers injected patients with Botox and had them complete a questionnaire that included questions on swallowing function after injection. Researchers also conducted various swallowing evaluation tests for an objective evaluation of swallowing. All five patients had improved swallowing that lasted from two to fourteen months; four had long-term improvement. Proof of the injection's benefits included a reduction in aspiration symptoms, an ability to eat solid foods, and weight gain. The injections did not cause any complications. Although the study size was small, the authors concluded that botulinum injection to treat dysphagia is effective when the cause is due to muscle spasm or hypertonicity.[1]

Japanese researchers reported on a patient case study in the potentially dangerous situation of undiagnosed dysphagia, which the researchers called *symptomless dysphagia* and which is also known as silent aspiration. Without obvious symptoms, the risk for aspiration pneumonia is greatly increased. The authors used the videofluoroscopy swallowing examination and a simple two-step swallowing provocation test (STS-SPT). They inserted technetium tin colloid (99mTc), a radionuclide, into a catheter placed in the patient's mouth as he slept. Radionuclides are isotopes that will appear on an X ray or videofluoroscopy. The following day the video image detected the symptomless dysphagia. In addition, the test resulted in improvement of the symptomless dysphagia. The authors believe that the 99mTc test may be particularly useful in detecting symptomless dysphagia in elderly stroke patients and could prevent the occurrence of aspiration pneumonia.[2]

In an effort to better understand the optimal diet and treatment for patients with dysphagia after a stroke, researchers reviewed studies with varying approaches as to how, when, and what to feed these patients. In addition to reviewing the medical databases, the authors contacted stroke researchers and equipment manufacturers. They limited their review to studies meeting specific criteria and that included dysphagic patients who had had a stroke within a specific three-month period. They found that if a patient needed to be fed through a tube (enteral nutrition), there was less risk for death if a percutaneous endoscopic gastrostomy (PEG) was used rather than a nasogastric tube (NGT). The NGT involves a thin, flexible feeding tube entered through the nose and residing in the stomach. With a PEG, a small incision is made on the abdominal surface and a tube is pulled through the nose to the stomach. The tube is then pulled through the incision; the end is anchored internally, but the tube itself is external. Use of a PEG tube also improved nutritional status, as measured by weight and other parameters, in this review. Swallowing therapy and drugs (nifedipine) did not appear to be beneficial. One trial reported that death was decreased when nutritional supplements were used, but the effect was not statistically significant. Supplements did, however, increase both energy and protein intake. The authors concluded that not enough studies have been done and that those that have been done had not included enough patients.[3]

Treatment and Nutritional Intervention

Historically, the diet for dysphagia was essentially a liquid diet. This recommendation did not change until clinicians realized that because dysphagia had many different causes, texture and consistency need to be altered in different ways for different patients. In fact, liquids are often more difficult to swallow than other forms of food, especially for most people with dysphagia. The next and most recent popularized regimen was the five-stage dysphagia diet, which consisted of progressing the diet from mostly liquid consistency to soft solids. The focus today is on individualizing the diet and relying on a swallowing evaluation to determine which textures and consistencies present the most problems for each patient. See Figure 3.3.

Because liquids are typically difficult to swallow, special commercial thickening agents can be useful in helping people with dysphagia to swallow and also to prevent dehydration. These thickeners can be added to liquids and foods. The swallowing evaluation provides information on the consistency that works best for each person: honey, nectar, or pudding thickness. In addition to special thickeners, baby rice cereal can work well to thicken foods. Although most patients can swallow thickened liquids better, some with dysphagia can handle thin liquids best.

- Avoid high-risk aspiration foods such as popcorn, bran cereal, nuts, fruit and vegetables with skin or fibrous pulp, corn, and celery.
- Avoid sticky foods such as fresh white bread, peanut butter, mashed potatoes without gravy, bananas, and refried beans.
- Divide meals into small, frequent feedings.
- Keep track of food intake and body weight; be alert for weight loss.
- If using pureed foods, be sure they are blended well (smooth, thick), not thin and watery.
- Include cold foods at meals to improve swallowing.
- Include highly seasoned, flavorful foods (they stimulate both appetite and the swallowing mechanism).
- To help prevent constipation, add bran to foods and consume adequate fluids.
- Use a standard vitamin–mineral supplement (providing 100 percent of the recommended daily allowances) to ensure adequate nutrient intake.

Figure 3.3 Dietary Recommendations for Dysphagia

Another helpful tip is to divide the meal pattern into small, frequent meals. Other aspects of food itself that can help swallowing include a cold temperature of food, carbonation, and sauces and gravies that lubricate foods. If the range of foods that the person with dysphagia can tolerate is narrow, it's wise to add a standard vitamin and mineral supplement. Constipation is a common problem because of the limited range of foods, especially those that contain fiber. Adding bran to foods and ensuring adequate fluid intake can help to prevent constipation.

In addition to careful assessment of foods that can be tolerated, it is important for dysphagia patients to eat and allow for extra time for meals. Keeping track of adequate food intake and body weight can help prevent weight loss and nutrient deficiencies. If swallowing is extremely weak and food intake is poor or if the risk for aspiration is high, however, it may be necessary to use nutrition support, specifically a tube feeding. Such support can be done during the night when the patient is sleeping; this method allows more freedom of movement during the day and encourages appetite and hunger sensations. If aspiration is a major concern, it is best to provide the tube feeding past the stomach and into the small intestine, where the risk is nonexistent. If the tube feeding continues beyond a few weeks, it is important to use an entry point other than the nose. Some people may object to a tube feeding because of the emotional and physical effects it can have. Thus, such a decision should be made carefully.

ACHALASIA

Achalasia is a condition in which nerve and muscle control in the esophagus is abnormal, which causes problems with peristalsis and opening of the lower esophageal sphincter (LES). A person with achalasia experiences difficulty swallowing and food not getting into the stomach as it should. This problem causes pain in the esophagus as it enlarges to accommodate swallowed food that remains in the esophagus too long. The condition can strike people of any age, even children, but it tends to develop between the ages of twenty and forty. At first, the symptoms are almost not noticeable, but the condition progresses over a period of months to a year.

Achalasia causes the same complications as dysphagia: choking, silent aspiration, and pneumonia. As with another condition involving the esophagus, gastroesophageal reflux disorder, achalasia increases the risk for esophageal cancer, with about 5 percent of people with achalasia developing such cancer. Physicians use the same tests for dysphagia to diagnose achalasia. The symptoms include pain in the esophagus, regurgitation, vomiting, indigestion, and weight loss. People with achalasia become afraid to eat because of the pain with which it's associated. Between this pain and other symptoms such as vomiting, nutritional status can become compromised.

Treatment

Treatment begins with changes in diet (see Figures 3.4 and 3.5). Most of the measures are geared to reducing the amount of food eaten at one time and avoiding foods that may be more likely to become stuck

---

Avoid the following foods only if they aggravate swallowing—eat bland foods if preferred:

- Bony fish
- Dry or crisp foods
- Excessively sweet drinks or fruits
- Foods that aggravate drooling
- Fibrous meats
- Sticky peanut butter or bananas
- Tart juices and foods
- Thinly pureed foods

Dietary/behavior modifications:

- Drink large volumes of fluid with each meal.
- Relax during meals; eat slowly and chew thoroughly.
- Eat small, frequent meals.
- Avoid extremes in food temperature.
- Elevate the head of the bed for thirty to forty-five minutes after meals and at bedtime.

Figure 3.4 Dietary Recommendations for Achalasia

Breakfast
- ¾   cup Cream of Wheat
- 2   teaspoons butter
- 1   cup 2 percent milk
- ½   cup apple juice
        coffee
- ½   ounce dairy creamer

Snack
- ½   cup pudding

Lunch
- 1   cup cream of chicken soup
- 1   dinner roll
- 1   teaspoon butter
- 1   cup 2 percent milk

Snack
- ½   cup applesauce
- ½   cup 2 percent cottage cheese

Dinner
- 4   ounces Salisbury steak, chopped or pureed
- ¼   cup gravy
- ½   cup mashed potatoes
- ½   cup creamed spinach
- ½   cup raspberry gelatin
- ½   cup grape juice
        iced tea

Snack
- 1   cup fruit yogurt

Calories 2,001; protein 77 g (15%); fat 72 g (32%); carbohydrate 274 g (53%); cholesterol 174 mg; calcium 1,594 mg; sodium 4,831 mg.

Figure 3.5 Sample Menu for Achalasia

in the esophagus and those most likely to irritate the delicate mucosa as they remain in contact with it longer than is normal.

Surgery may become necessary if dietary measures can't manage the achalasia and especially if food intake decreases significantly, making the patient malnourished. One type of procedure widens the sphincter and forces it to open by inflating a balloon placed down through the esophagus. This method works for about 40 percent of people with the disorder, although they may need the dilation procedure repeated. A new and intriguing treatment, injection of botulinum toxin into the LES, is showing promising results, as effective as the dilation procedure (see the research update section later in this chapter). Experts say that more research is needed to see the long-term effects, both for effectiveness and safety. When both of these methods fail, a surgeon must cut the muscle fibers in the LES. The success rate for this surgery is 85 percent, but about 15 percent of patients will have reflux as a result.

GASTROESOPHAGEAL REFLUX DISEASE (GERD)

Most of us have had heartburn, an unpleasant burning sensation coming up into the throat, often bringing with it discomfort in the chest area and thus earning its name. When infrequent, heartburn is a relatively normal occurrence. For many people, heartburn occurs if they exert themselves too soon after eating a full meal or overindulge in high-fat foods and alcohol; it can even occur in rhythm with female hormones, either during the week before a menstrual cycle or in pregnancy. The medical term for heartburn is gastroesophageal reflux, which is a bit more descriptive of the process in which acid from the stomach refluxes up into the esophagus. The resultant inflammation of the sensitive tissue of the esophagus, which isn't protected from acid as is the stomach, is called *esophagitis*. Acute esophagitis can be caused by ingesting a caustic compound such as a particular medication; 20 percent of people who routinely take nonsteroidal anti-inflammatory drugs, such as aspirin or ibuprofen, develop esophagitis. It can also occur with repeated vomiting, especially when the vomiting is self-induced, as in bulimia.

For over 19 million Americans, the problem is chronic, and rather than random, infrequent episodes, it doesn't go away. At this point, it becomes a disease and is called *gastroesophageal reflux disorder*, or GERD. The exact cause of GERD is not clear, although various studies have pointed to risk factors such as obesity. Contributing factors behind GERD include a high amount of acid in the stomach; looseness of the LES, which separates the stomach and the esophagus; motility problems of the esophagus causing abnormal peristaltic waves; and a slow rate of gastric emptying. In GERD, the LES opens when it should stay closed, allowing stomach acid to enter the esophagus. Many factors affect the pressure of the sphincter and therefore its opening and closing. These factors include hormones; nutrients; medications; high abdominal pressure as with chronic lung disease; lying down after meals; and substances such as caffeine, mint, cigarettes, alcohol, and chocolate (see Table 3.1 and Figure 3.6).

Symptoms and Diagnosis

The general symptoms of GERD include a burning sensation in the throat, difficulty swallowing, and tightness or pain in the chest area just behind the breastbone, but they can also include coughing, shortness of breath, and even vomiting of blood. The specific symptoms and their severity depend on the acidity (which diet can influence) and the amount of the reflux and on how often it occurs. If it's frequent and the symptoms are severe, the esophagus can become ulcerated, leading to the formation of scar tissue that narrows the opening

Table 3.1 Factors Affecting Lower Esophageal Sphincter Pressure in Gastroesophageal Reflux Disease

Reduce Pressure (Open)	*Increase Pressure (Close)*
Alcoholic beverages	Dietary protein
Caffeine	
Chocolate	*Medications*
Cigarettes	Bethanecol
Dietary fat	Metoclopropamide
Mint oils	

High Pressure on stomach
  Overeating, drinking

Hormone level
  Progesterone (pregnancy, late phase of menstrual cycle)

Medications
  Anticholinergics: Atropine, Bentyl, Robinul, scopolamine
  Bronchodilators: Albuterol (Proventil, Ventolin); metaproterenol
  (Alupent); montelukast (Singulair); terbutaline (Brethine); theophylline
  (Aerolate, Slo-Bid, Slo-Phyllin, Theo-24, Theo-Dur, Theolair, Uniphyl);
  zafirlukast (Accolate)

and makes swallowing more difficult. In addition, as the ulcerated tissue bleeds, often before some people seek treatment, anemia can develop. GERD also significantly increases the risk for a precancerous condition called Barrett's esophagus. A person experiencing frequent and severe GERD may be afraid to eat because of pain, which usually leads to weight loss and nutrient deficiencies. Because of these possible complications, a person with symptoms should not take chronic heartburn lightly.

The tests that physicians use to diagnose GERD are similar to those for dysphagia (see Figure 3.2 on page 31). These tests provide information on LES pressure, acid reflux, and the person's ability to clear acid from the esophagus. The last test is important because GERD

Medications
- **Calcium channel blockers:** Adalat, Calan, Cardene, Cardizem, DynaCirc, Isoptin, Nimotop, Norvasc, Plendil, Posicor, Procardia, Sular, Vascor, Verelan

- **Opiates/opioids:** Alfenta, Buprenex, codeine, Dalgan, Darvon, Demerol, Dilaudid, Dolophine, Levo-Dromoran, Nubain, Roxicodone, Sublimaze, Sufenta, Talwin, Ultiva

- **Tricyclic antidepressants:** Adapin/Sinequan, Anafranil Aventyl/Pamelor, Janimine/Tofranil, Vivactil, Norpramin/Pertofrane

Other Substances
- Alcohol

- Marijuana

- Tobacco

Figure 3.6 Substances That Slow Gastric Emptying

causes inflammation of the esophagus, which in turn compromises swallowing ability. In addition, Bernstein's test, also called acid perfusion, can help to determine if the symptom of pain is caused by acid reflux. In this test, hydrochloric acid is introduced into the esophagus, and if the person experiences pain, it means that acid reflux is causing their pain. If there is no pain, reflux is not the problem.

Another test for GERD is the gastroesophageal reflux scan, also called GE reflux and aspiration scan. Besides helping to diagnose GERD, this scan also provides feedback on the effectiveness of treatment and detects aspiration of stomach contents into the lungs. For the GE reflux scan, the patient lies down and then swallows a tracer cocktail. The cocktail contains orange juice, weak hydrochloric acid, and a radionuclide, a radio-opaque compound that allows it to appear on an X ray. The technician takes X-ray images over the length of the esophagus and then asks the patient to assume various positions to determine if reflux occurs and, if so, in which position. Next, the technician places an inflatable cuff around the patient's abdomen, similar to those used on the arm for measuring blood pressure. As the cuff is inflated, abdominal pressure increases and more images are taken over the esophagus to see if reflux occurs.

Another useful test is the gastric emptying scan, which is similar in nature to the GE reflux scan. This test determines the time it takes for the contents of the stomach, usually food, to leave the stomach and enter the small intestine; a typical time is 90 to 120 minutes. The gastric emptying scan can be useful in determining the underlying problem in GERD, because if food stays too long in the stomach it's more likely that some, along with stomach acid, will reflux up into the esophagus. In this test, the patient eats a light meal containing a radionuclide, and the technician scans the stomach until gastric emptying is complete. In addition to contributing to GERD, delayed gastric emptying is a common consequence of tumors or other obstructions near the lower opening of the stomach and of various medications and substances. Other causes of obstruction include scarring and edema, which can arise from ulcers in the duodenum; diabetes; and disorders of the nervous system.

Research Update on GERD

Obesity was once considered a contributing factor to GERD, but the role of obesity in the pathogenesis of gastroesophageal reflux, as well as the benefit of weight loss, has not been proven.[4] Tight-fitting clothes, which may be worn by obese individuals, may increase the risk of reflux. Researchers who tested the hypothesis that weight reduction improves the manifestations of gastroesophageal reflux found no reduction in reflux according to pH measurement and no significant changes in reflux symptoms.[5]

Researchers studied participants in the first National Health and Nutrition Examination Survey and examined the relationship of weight, dietary fat intake, and other factors with reflux disease hospitalization.[6] Patients were followed an average of eighteen and a half years. The researchers found a correlation between high reflux disease hospitalization rates and a patient's high body mass index (BMI). No relationship was found between higher fat intake and reflux disease hospitalization. Other factors associated with reflux disease hospitalization included age, low recreational activity, and a history of doctor-diagnosed arthritis.

Another study determined whether obesity is associated with the presence of a hiatal hernia or diagnosis of esophagitis.[7] A retrospective case control study used patients who had undergone gastric analysis and upper GI endoscopy between 1974 and 1995. Excessive body weight was significantly associated with the presence of hiatal hernia as well as with esophagitis. When controlled for the effect of hiatal hernia, the association between BMI and esophagitis diminished but remained significant. The authors concluded that excessive body weight is a significant independent risk factor for hiatal hernia and is significantly associated with esophagitis, largely through the increased incidence of hiatal hernia.

Helicobacter pylori (H. pylori) is a common infection, largely responsible for chronic gastritis and gastroduodenal ulcer disease. Its relation to gastroesophageal reflux disease (GERD), however, has not yet been well established.[8] Available data suggest that the infection is not a risk factor for the disease and could even characterize a protective factor. Epidemiological studies have shown that patients with GERD have similar incidence rates of *H. pylori* infection as do control groups.[9] Some data show an even lower incidence, leading researchers to deduce that infection does not cause, and in some way may reduce the risk of, GERD.[10] Supportive evidence shows the development of GERD following successful *H. pylori* elimination, and *H. pylori* infection has been found to be negatively correlated with the severity of esophagitis. The mechanisms are complicated.[11]

Previous studies have shown proton pump inhibitors (PPIs), which decrease acid secretion, are more effective in *H. pylori*–positive individuals.[12] On the downside, some reports suggest that *H. pylori* infection and PPI treatment increase an individual's risk of developing gastric atrophy.[13] Atrophic gastritis is considered a risk factor for the subsequent development of gastric cancer.

One treatment strategy based on these issues is *H. pylori* treatment given to patients with GERD requiring medications such as PPIs. However, the Canadian consensus report does not currently support this management strategy, as there is a need for additional supportive evidence to link *H. pylori* and the long-term use of PPIs with the development of gastric atrophy.[14]

GERD patients are commonly advised by their doctors to avoid fatty foods,[15] yet there is minimal data to support the effectiveness of such a regimen. Results of recent studies have shown no confirmation.

Researchers in Italy measured the acidity and pressures of the esophagus for three hours after a high-fat and a typical balanced meal.[16] The high-fat meal contained 52 percent fat, and the balanced meal contained 24 percent fat. Eight controls and seven patients were studied in both lying down and sitting positions. The high-fat meal did not increase the rate of reflux episodes or alter LES motor function in either group, regardless of body position.

In contrast, one experimental study found that when compared with a salt and water solution, the infusion of a solution containing only fat into the small intestine caused a modest increase in the number of reflux episodes in patients with reflux esophagitis.[17] This observation, however, is unrealistic in the practical sense because it is unlikely that a person will consume 100 percent fat in a meal.

Despite these results, a low-fat diet should not be ruled out in patients with gastroesophageal reflux. Other hypotheses remain to be tested with longer observation periods.[18] The possibility exists that a higher fat content delays gastric emptying and consequently increases reflux hours after a meal. Regardless of studies done, some patients report that fatty foods are not well accepted. Individual tolerances are extremely important in deciding what is best for a patient.

Treatment and Nutritional Intervention

Treatment for GERD can include diet and lifestyle changes, medications, and, failing these, surgery. Dietary considerations for GERD focus on three objectives: prevent pain and irritation in the esophagus during a flare-up, prevent reflux, and lower the acidity of the stomach's contents (see Figure 3.7). Achieving these objectives involves manipulating dietary aspects that affect LES pressure and therefore whether the LES opens or stays closed, reducing gastric acid secretion, and avoiding tart or acidic foods and irritating spices during a flare-up. During a flare-up, the esophageal membranes are inflamed and sensitive, and it may be helpful to consume a liquid (avoiding citrus juices, which are acidic). As food intake becomes possible, it is best to avoid spices such as chili powder or black pepper, which may irritate the tissue. In addition, crispy, dry, and fibrous foods such as certain types of crackers and raw vegetables may physically irritate an inflamed esophagus.

To prevent or reduce the frequency of reflux, the emphasis should be on avoiding foods that lower LES pressure, causing it to open inappropriately (see Table 3.1 on page 41). In addition, small, frequent meals may be useful; the smaller the amount of food in the stomach, the less likely it is to increase abdominal pressure on the LES sphincter. Another

Diet to Prevent Reflux

- Eat small, frequent meals; avoid large meals.

- Avoid single high-fat meals.

- Eat low-fat, higher protein meals.

- Limit alcohol.

- Avoid foods that lower LES pressure, such as chocolate, coffee, mints, garlic, onions, and cinnamon. (Base consumption of garlic, onions, and cinnamon on individual experience.)

- Avoid drinking liquids with meals; drink between meals.

Other Aspects of Treatment

- Do not lie down after eating; wait at least three hours.

- Elevate the head of the bed, if needed.

- Limit or avoid smoking.

- Use antacids to lower gastric acidity (read product labels carefully).

Diet for Acute Esophagitis (inflamed, irritated)

- Avoid acidic foods (citrus fruits, tomatoes).

- Avoid spicy foods (red pepper, black pepper).

- Follow a bland, soft diet.

- Eat small, frequent meals.

Figure 3.7 Dietary Recommendations for Gastroesophageal Reflux Disease

tip is to avoid drinking liquids with a meal; rather, consume beverages one hour before a meal, reducing the amount of the stomach contents at any one time and preventing high abdominal pressure.

Along with diet, some lifestyle changes may also help. Some studies have implicated obesity as a risk factor, although other studies have refuted such findings. Wearing tight-fitting clothes, especially in the abdominal area, appears to increase the chance for reflux. People who enjoy lying down after eating may want to change their habits if GERD is a problem, mostly because of the shift in pressure toward the sphincter and the assistance of gravity. The same advice goes for people who eat a large meal late in the evening and head for bed soon after. A waiting period of about three hours between a meal and bedtime is optimal.

Lowering the acidity of the stomach is important because in the event of a reflux episode, the liquid refluxing from the stomach will cause less pain and irritation if the stomach's acid level is lower. Some substances—coffee (both decaffeinated and regular), fermented alcoholic beverages such as wine and beer, and cigarette smoke—cause an increase in acid secretion, so it's best to avoid them. Smoking exerts a wide range of GI effects, most of which worsen GI problems (see Figure 3.8). The most effective way to reduce gastric acidity is to use antacids (see Table 3.2 and Figure 3.9). To maximize their acid-lowering effect, these drugs should be taken about one to three hours after a meal. Antacids and good intentions, however, won't fix this recipe for GERD disaster: washing down a high-fat meal of spicy beef

- Increases acid secretion
- Reduces lower esophageal sphincter pressure (opens)
- Inhibits bicarbonate secretion from pancreas
- Increases gastric emptying of liquids
- Increases acidity in duodenum
- Interferes with the action of some GI drugs
- Impairs healing of ulcers

Figure 3.8 Effects of Smoking on the Gastrointestinal System

Table 3.2 Medications for Gastroesophageal Reflux Disease (GERD)

Antacids	*Trade Name*
Aluminum hydroxide	Amphojel, Alternagel,* Dialume
Calcium carbonate	Tums
Magnesium hydroxide	Uro-Mag, Phillips Milk of Magnesia
Combinations of above	Gelusil*, Maalox, Mylanta II*
Magaldrate	Riopan*
GI Stimulants	
Metoclopramide	Reglan
Cisapride	Propulsid
H2 Receptor Antagonists/ *Proton Pump Inhibitors*	
Cimetidine	Tagamet
Famotidine	Pepcid
Lansoprazole	Prevacid
Nizatidine	Axid
Omeprazole	Prilosec
Ranitidine	Zantac

*Also contains simethicone.

enchiladas with a beer, capping it off with a gooey chocolate dessert and coffee, smoking a cigarette, and then going off to bed.

If diet changes don't improve GERD, medications are the next step. If after six months the drugs are unsuccessful, which is true in up to 10 percent of patients, a few surgical procedures are available. The traditional surgical technique is fundoplication, in which the surgeon wraps the fundus of the stomach around the lower esophagus.

An intriguing new procedure, endo lumenal gastroplication, may help some GERD sufferers toss their medications and may even prevent the need for more invasive surgery.[19] Instead of surgery or placing objects in the esophagus, this procedure uses an endoscope to put

Breakfast
  2   cups Cheerios
  1   cup 1 percent milk
  1   cup apple juice

Lunch
  1   4-ounce veggie burger patty
  1   hamburger bun
  2   cups tossed salad
  2   tablespoons dressing
  1   cup low-fat fruit yogurt
  1   cup grape juice

Dinner
  1   6-ounce roasted chicken breast
  1   cup pasta salad
  1   cup steamed broccoli
  1   cup 1 percent milk
  1   peach

Snack
  1   ounce string cheese
  4–5 carrot sticks

Calories 1,969; protein 108 g (22%); fat 55 g (25%); carbohydrate 281 g (53%); calcium 1,634 mg; cholesterol 143 mg.

Figure 3.9 Sample Menu for Gastroesophageal Reflux Disease

a few stitches in the LES, which prevents acid from seeping up from the stomach into the esophagus. The FDA has approved the procedure, and a few major medical centers around the country are already performing it. Aside from the obvious benefit of not having surgery, endo lumenal gastroplication only takes an hour to perform and costs one-third less than fundoplication. Researchers said that eight medical centers performing the procedure reported that 70 percent of patients were able to significantly reduce their use of anti-GERD medications.[20] Some GERD patients, however, are not good candidates for endo lumenal gastroplication, including those who have had stomach surgery and those with precancerous conditions or dysphagia.

HIATAL HERNIA

Hiatal hernia, a common cause of reflux, consists of an outpouching of part of the stomach up through the opening of the diaphragm (see Figure 3.10). The opening of the diaphragm normally accommodates the esophagus, but in a hiatal hernia, the stomach extrudes through it as well. This extrusion exerts pressure on the LES, which opens when it should remain closed. The result is often gastro-

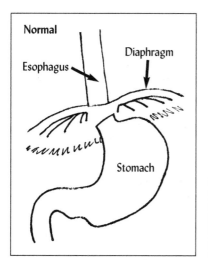
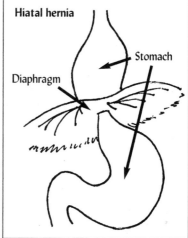

Figure 3.10 (*Left*) Normal position of the esophagus, diaphragm, and stomach; (*Right*) Hiatal hernia

esophageal reflux with the same symptoms as GERD. Different types of hiatal hernias may develop, and the form of the outpouching gives the condition its name.

The most common type, representing 90 percent of all cases, is the sliding hiatal hernia. With this condition, part of the stomach and the LES herniate through the diaphragm. Many people experience mild or even no symptoms, and experts estimate that up to 40 percent of Americans have a sliding hiatal hernia and don't know it. Another type of hiatel hernia is the paraesophageal hiatal hernia, in which the outpouching extrudes through the diaphragm and sits next to the esophagus. Because the LES remains in the normal position, the paraesophageal hiatal hernia produces no symptoms. It can, however, get trapped or pinched by the diaphragm, resulting in a serious situation called strangulation that requires immediate surgery. Although rare, both types of hernias can bleed from their lining, either tiny amounts that can lead to anemia or life-threatening massive bleeding.

The cause of most cases of hiatal hernia is not known, but injury or trauma can produce the problem. One theory suggests that unexplained cases may be the result of a congenital shortening of the GI tract. The person with the defect may not develop a hiatal hernia until later in life, with the onset occurring as a result of some type of stress. In women, it may be the physiologic stress of pregnancy. For both men and women, extreme physical exertion may trigger the hiatal hernia.

Symptoms and Diagnosis

Not all people with a sliding hiatal hernia experience reflux, but for most, that is the major symptom. Some people with hiatal hernia may have difficulty breathing when they lie down or bend over. Others feel pain in the upper region of the stomach after eating a large meal, especially one that is high in fat. Diagnosis of hiatal hernia is straightforward, because it appears on a standard X ray. The physician, however, may have to press rather forcefully on the abdomen to detect the sliding hiatal hernia.

Research Update on Hiatal Hernia

Researchers have suggested several mechanisms that may cause GERD, including hiatal hernia, failure of extrinsic diaphragmatic compression of the esophagus, weak basal lower esophageal sphincter (LES) pressure, and transient LES relaxations.[21] The link between hiatal hernia and GERD is controversial. Several studies, however, have shown that 50 to 94 percent of patients with GERD have a hiatal hernia, with a significantly lower percentage in control subjects.[22]

A study by Kahrilas et al. found that hiatal hernia reduces LES pressure and alters its responsiveness. This study measured the intraluminal pressure profile of patients with hiatal hernia and of normal subjects. They found that by altering the pressures of the connection between the esophagus and stomach, hiatal hernia may increase susceptibility to reflux associated with diminished LES pressure. Other scientists had concerns about the methods used in this experiment.[23] Still, most researchers agree that hiatal hernia is important in the development of GERD.[24] Many factors may be involved in the development of GERD, and they may vary among individuals.[25] Recent studies still support hiatal hernia as a contributor to GERD.

A familial occurrence of hiatal hernia was first suggested in 1949.[26] Since then, familial occurrence of sliding hiatal hernia has been reported in more than twenty cases.[27] The pattern of inheritance of hiatal hernia has been documented only rarely. In the largest investigation to date, thirty-eight members of a family across five generations were analyzed.[28] Family members were interviewed and investigated for hiatal hernia by a barium swallow; of thirty-eight family members, twenty-three had evidence of a hiatal hernia. No individual with a hiatal hernia was born to unaffected parents. This study found familial inheritance of hiatal hernia does occur. In one case, direct male-to-male transmission was shown between father and son.

Treatment

The dietary approach for hiatal hernia is the same as for GERD: keep abdominal pressure low and prevent reflux.

CHAPTER 4

Diseases of the Stomach and Duodenum

■ · · · · · · ■

GASTRITIS

Gastritis is a gastrointestinal disease with a simple definition: inflammation and damage of the lining of the stomach. The damage occurs when the uppermost mucosal layer, which protects the stomach from its own corrosive acid and enzymes, becomes eroded and exposes underlying tissue to these digestive juices. This erosion can arise from several sources, but recent research has shown that the bacteria *Helicobacter pylori* is responsible for the majority of gastritis and ulcer cases. The development of gastritis is serious; it can be life threatening in and of itself, but it also increases the risk of stomach ulcers and cancer. In addition, nutritional health can become compromised because of poor food intake, vomiting, and nutrient absorption problems.

The story behind *H. pylori* is a fascinating tale of detective work and outright bravery. Researchers had speculated for some time that a bacterium might be responsible for gastritis and peptic ulcer disease (PUD). A couple of Australian researchers in the early 1980s turned speculation into fact. Believing that a bug was the cause of PUD but unable to prove it, a young gastroenterologist, Barry Marshall, decided to gulp down a sample of a suspected bacterium. Within weeks, he developed severe stomach pains and looked for all the world as a person suffering from gastritis, yet the severe gastritis vanished without any treatment.

A few years later, another Australian who ingested an *H. pylori* cocktail wasn't as fortunate as Marshall. He showed signs of infection for only ten days, but the infection persisted. On the sixty-seventh day, he took Pepto-Bismol (bismuth subsalicylate). About a month later, a biopsy showed that the treatment had cured the gastritis, but nine months later, another biopsy showed that the infection and the gastritis had returned. He had to be treated with two different antibiotics to eradicate the infection, a process that took three years. After that, researchers began in earnest to study the bug and its link to gastritis and ulcer. Today, thanks to the volumes of scientific studies, much more is known about *H. pylori* (see Figure 4.1). Some mysteries still remain, however, not the least of which is why some people who are infected, such as Marshall, do not develop chronic gastritis.

H. pylori grows in the mucus-secreting cells of the stomach lining. It is the only known bacteria that can survive and grow in the stomach's acidic environment. Interestingly, the human stomach is the only place these bugs have been found. Although *H. pylori* is the culprit in most cases and represents a chronic form of gastritis, many other factors can also cause gastritis. Acute gastritis is caused by ingestion of mucosal irritants, which could either be an accidental ingestion of a caustic chemical or chronic use of certain drugs. Another type of acute gastritis, acute stress gastritis, is caused by injury or sudden illness.

Types of Gastritis

There are many different types of gastritis.

Acute gastritis is caused by ingestion of corrosive compounds or receiving high-dose radiation.

Q What is *Helicobacter pylori*?

A *H. pylori* is a corkscrew-shaped microscopic bacterial organism. It lives in the mucous layer of the human stomach.

Q How do you get infected?

A Scientists are not certain how a person gets *H. pylori*, but like most infections, it is spread from one person to another. Methods of transmission include using unsterilized diagnostic equipment, such as an endoscope, eating contaminated food, and drinking contaminated water.

Q What does the infection do to a person?

A Not everyone who is infected develops a disease. Diseases associated with *H. pylori* include gastritis, stomach cancer, peptic ulcer disease, and possibly gastroesophageal reflux disease.

Q How many people have the infection?

A Experts say that in less developed countries where sanitation and hygiene are poor, the infection rate may be as high as 90 percent. The world average is 66 percent. In the United States, the rate is 25 percent, and high-risk groups include the elderly, African Americans, Hispanics, and people with limited resources.

Q How does a person know if he or she is infected?

A A blood test can show *H. pylori* antibodies, indicating possible infection. In addition, a breath test, in which a person is given a special drink that measures carbon dioxide production, can show the bug's presence. Other more invasive methods include biopsy and tissue culture.

Q What is the best way to protect against *H. pylori*?

A Scientists still are not sure, so at this point the best protection includes frequent and proper hand-washing; drinking water only from clean, safe sources; and using proper sanitation techniques in food preparation.

Figure 4.1 Common Questions About *Helicobacter pylori*

Acute stress gastritis is a severe type of gastritis caused by a sudden illness or injury, the latter of which need not be to the stomach. Most often, acute stress gastritis is caused by extensive burns and injuries that cause significant bleeding. Other disease states that can cause acute stress gastritis include high fever, heart attack, and kidney failure.

Atrophic gastritis is a form of gastritis that occurs when antibodies attack the stomach lining, causing it to become very thin and lose all or many of the cells that produce acid and enzymes. This condition usually affects elderly people, but it also can occur in those who have had part of the stomach removed (partial gastrectomy). Atrophic gastritis can cause pernicious anemia, the deficiency of B_{12}, and iron-deficiency anemia because of the low acid conditions.

Chronic erosive gastritis is a gradually developing type of gastritis arising from ingestion of drugs that irritate the stomach's lining; from alcohol abuse, which has the same effect; from Crohn's disease, an inflammatory disease of the small intestine; and from bacterial or viral infections. The most common drug-induced gastritis is caused by chronic use of nonsteroidal anti-inflammatory drugs (NSAIDs) (see Figure 4.2).

Ménétrier's disease is gastritis with an unknown cause in which the walls of the stomach form thick folds, enlarged glands, and cysts. The disorder increases risk for stomach cancer.

Plasma cell gastritis is a type of gastritis with an unknown cause in which white blood cells (plasma cells) accumulate in various organs and in the stomach wall.

Viral or fungal gastritis is a form of gastritis that develops in patients during or after a long illness or in those with deficient immune systems.

Although *H. pylori* is somewhat resistant to the stomach's acid, it is not immune. It protects itself in two ways: by hiding beneath the protective mucosal layer and by secreting the enzyme urease. Urease promotes ammonia formation to neutralize the acidity of the bacteria's immediate surroundings. Experts say that infection rates are close to 50 percent of the population in developed countries and 90 percent in less developed nations. The difference in infection between

Aleve/Anaprox	Feldene	Orudis
aspirin	Indocin	Relafen
Ansaid	Lodine	sodium salicylate
Arthropan	mesalamine	Tolectin
Clinoril	Motrin	Toradol
Daypro	Nalfon	Voltaren
Dolobid	Naprosyn	

Figure 4.2 Nonsteroidal Anti-Inflammatory Drugs (NSAIDs)

developed and less developed countries may be related to less sanitary conditions and poor hygiene in some parts of the world. In the United States, experts have estimated that 25 percent of Americans are infected with *H. pylori*.[1] With these high infection rates, it's not clear why only 10 to 15 percent of those infected develop gastritis or ulcers.

The difference between merely having an infection and developing the disease is probably related to a person's genetic makeup and aspects of his or her environment and lifestyle. Prior to learning about *H. pylori,* researchers blamed gastritis and ulcers on these factors. Once the infection takes hold, the body mounts an immune response, causing a continual state of inflammation. In response to the inflammation, *H. pylori* secretes toxins that damage the stomach. The damage may begin as gastritis, but later it progresses to ulcers.

Symptoms and Diagnosis

Gastritis symptoms depend on the type or cause of the disease, but most people experience indigestion and pain in the upper abdomen. For example, acute stress gastritis develops quickly after the initial injury or illness, usually within a week. From there, the gastritis can progress to bruises, ulcers, and bleeding, which can be fatal. Symptoms associated with GI bleeding include melena (black, tarry stools) and vomiting. The vomiting is called coffee ground emesis because the regurgitated matter of partially digested blood resembles that familiar by-product. Other gastritis symptoms include nausea, heartburn, loss of appetite, and weight loss.

Diagnostic procedures include endoscopy, in this case a gastroscopy because the scope is going into the stomach, and biopsy of stomach tissue in which a sample of tissue is removed for study. With endoscopy, the physician can actually see the lining of the stomach and can detect inflammation or ulceration. Using the endoscope, the physician can also take a biopsy and stop bleeding by cauterizing damaged areas. A biopsy will show the presence of *H. pylori,* as will a blood test in which antibodies to the bacteria appear after infection.

Research Update on Gastritis

Japanese researchers wanting to know if eating specific foods was associated with *H. pylori* infection conducted a study of 365 subjects, 104 men and 261 women, in an area with a high rate of *H. pylori* infection. The researchers randomly selected subjects from over 7,000 inhabitants over the age of twenty. They found antibodies to the bacteria in 83.7 percent of the population, with higher rates in older people. Subjects with gastritis, peptic ulcer, and cancer were more often infected than those without those diseases. Smoking, drinking habits, and gender were not associated with *H. pylori* infection. The daily intake of cereals, potatoes and starches, and milk was higher in infected subjects, but those who drank tea and ate algae were infected less often. The intake of the essential mineral zinc was higher in people with *H. pylori.* In contrast, people with higher iron intake were less likely to be infected. The researchers believe that the dietary intake of zinc and iron may affect the possibility of becoming infected with *H. pylori*.[2]

When children develop stomach or duodenal ulcers or gastritis, it is often as a result of trauma, Crohn's disease, or medications, especially NSAIDs. When they develop chronic gastritis or ulcers that are not caused by these conditions, however, it is almost always due to *H. pylori* infection.[3]

Treatment and Nutritional Intervention

If the gastritis is due to *H. pylori* infection, treatment must include antibiotics (amoxicillin, clarithromycin), bismuth, and the antiulcer medication, omeprazole. Eradicating the *H. pylori* infection, however, sometimes proves challenging. In noninfectious gastritis caused by some type of irritating agent, such as NSAIDs or alcohol, it's important to avoid the offending substances. In addition, with most types of gastritis, antiulcer drugs and antacids are routine therapy because of their ability to shut down acid production and prevent further damage.

The nutrition care objectives and diet for gastritis depend on the type of gastritis: chronic, acute, or a flare-up of chronic gastritis (see Figure 4.3). In acute gastritis or a flare-up that sends the person to the hospital, it's important to not stimulate gastric secretions and to empty the stomach to allow healing of the mucosal lining. The patient will receive liquids to quench thirst, but no solid food, generally for twenty-four to forty-eight hours, depending on the severity of the attack. If the patient had poor appetite and weight loss prior to the attack, he or she may need parenteral nutrition. As healing occurs, the diet progresses to a soft or bland diet (see Table 4.1).

The soft diet for GI problems is a low-fiber diet that provides a transition from a liquid diet to a normal or regular diet. In contrast, the bland diet eliminates foods or substances that irritate the gastric mucosa. Aside from these broad descriptions, however, hospitals often

Acute Gastritis

- Drink only liquids for twenty-four to forty-eight hours.

- Omit alcohol.

- Omit lactose-containing products (dairy foods) if they cause problems.

- Progress to soft or bland diet as tolerated; gradually add fiber foods.

- Use parenteral nutrition if patient is compromised or if unable to feed for more than three days.

Chronic Gastritis

- Avoid alcohol.

- Omit lactose-containing products (dairy foods) if they cause problems.

- Avoid caffeine.

- Eat small, frequent meals.

- Eat a low-fat diet to promote proper gastric emptying.

Figure 4.3 Dietary Recommendations for Gastritis

interpret these diets quite differently. For example, some institutions eliminate fried foods from a bland diet. This practice was standard a few years back, but with the liberalization of the bland diet, it was thought to be unnecessary. A study in Italy, however, found that fried foods, independent of the total fat content, reduced gastric emptying.[4] By increasing the time it takes for food to leave the stomach, fried foods could aggravate gastritis and other digestive problems.

Gastritis can cause problems for specific nutrients, so it's important to assess the patient's nutrient status. Because chronic gastritis may reduce the stomach's secretions, vitamin B_{12} may need to be supplemented. In addition to acid and enzymes, the stomach's cells secrete the intrinsic factor, which is needed to absorb the B vitamin from food. Iron may be a problem if acid secretion is low, or if there has been a

Table 4.1 Diets for Stomach Disorders

Soft Diet	*Bland Diet*
Avoid	Avoid
Highly seasoned foods (see Bland Diet list)	Pepper, chili powder, curry powder, cocoa, chocolate (and food and beverages containing these)
Fried foods	
Tough foods	
Whole-grain products	Caffeine (and food and beverages containing any)
Nuts and seeds	
Most fresh fruits and vegetables	Regular and decaffeinated coffee
Pepper	Alcohol
Use	Use
Small, frequent meals	Individual tolerance in planning
Individual tolerance in planning	Regular meals; frequent meals not needed

chronic use of antacids. The normal acid level of the stomach changes the iron to a form that is more absorbable.

In Ménétrier's disease, also called hypertrophic gastritis, an important aspect of diet is to replace protein that is lost because of the disease. Following a high-protein diet will help to ensure that nutritional status doesn't become compromised. The extra protein probably is not that much, considering that most Americans eat much more protein than they need. The recommendation is for 20 percent of total energy to come from protein. For the average person needing 2,000 calories daily, that works out to adding an extra serving of protein to the typical meal pattern of up to 6 ounces of lean meat; three servings of low-fat dairy products; and a minimum of six servings of bread, cereal, or other grain.

PEPTIC ULCER DISEASE

Peptic ulcer disease (PUD) is the collective term for ulcers, which are eroded areas of tissue in either the stomach or the duodenum. The erosion arises from the stomach's own acid and protein-digesting enzyme, pepsin. The underlying tissue and nerves are exposed, causing severe pain. The majority of ulcers, about 85 percent of all cases in the United States, are duodenal, occurring in the first ten inches of the organ. Gastric ulcers tend to develop in the upper curve of the stomach. Just as the stress of severe illness or trauma can cause gastritis, it can also produce ulcers, appropriately named stress ulcers.

Although the prevalence of PUD has been declining for the past several years, the disease continues to take its toll, with over 25 million Americans suffering from an ulcer at some point in their lifetimes. Experts estimate that PUD costs Americans $6 billion for treatments and loss of work and productivity. The 1990s witnessed the advent of effective treatments for many people with PUD, but the disease can still cause life-threatening complications, including perforation, bleeding, and obstruction. Nutritionally, people with PUD often restrict their diet unnecessarily, which means that the intake of essential nutrients may be less than optimal. In addition, pain and other GI symptoms may affect food intake and may weaken nutritional health.

For many years, the cause of PUD was thought to involve a combination of weak host defenses, excess acid secretion, and damaging aspects of the diet. Extremely restrictive diets were the mainstay of treatment. As more research emerged, however, it became clear that food and drink did not have the power to cause or cure PUD. Acid is not the primary cause, but it is involved in some way, because its inhibition plays an important role in treatment. The only exception to the idea that acid is not the primary cause is a disease called *Zollinger-Ellison syndrome*, in which a tumor in the pancreas secretes gastrin, causing massive amounts of acid that produce ulceration to be released.

The breakthrough came in the 1990s with the discovery that *H. pylori* was the culprit responsible for half of all PUD. Scientists are still theorizing as to how the bacteria wreak their damage. As with gastritis, many people with *H. pylori* never develop PUD, which shows that other factors influence the disease. A person's genes are of special importance, because they dictate the amount of protective mucus secreted and the amount of tissue-eroding acid. Many studies have suggested that certain foods or nutrients may influence the development of PUD, but there are no clear answers. So far, a few studies have pointed to a possible protective effect of polyunsaturated fats, fiber, and vitamin A against developing PUD.[5]

Gastric ulcers are often the result of chronic use of medications that irritate the mucosa, such as NSAIDs. When a person stops using an NSAID, the ulcers heal and usually do not return. People with gastric ulcers tend to have normal to low acid levels, so the development probably involves weakened defenses. In contrast, about 66 percent of people with duodenal ulcers have a high level of acid secretion, even in a nonstimulated state such as fasting or sleeping. The excess acid is a result of having up to twice as many parietal cells, the cells that secrete acid, as the average person. The high acid content of the stomach normally moves into the duodenum, where it's neutralized by bicarbonate from the pancreas. For people with duodenal ulcers who are often secreting too much acid, the neutralizing effect can't keep up with the excess acid, which then erodes the tissue. It's important to note, however, that just as with *H. pylori* infection, many people have excess acid but don't develop ulcers.

Gastric ulcers tend to develop later in life, whereas duodenal ulcers can occur at any age. Onset may be related to the use of NSAIDs, which may be more typical for the elderly who experience chronic pain or inflammation with diseases such as arthritis. Of concern with gastric ulcers is that they increase the risk for stomach cancer and mortality. Duodenal ulcers, however, almost never develop into cancer.

The two types of PUD also differ in the symptoms they cause in people with the disease.

Symptoms and Diagnosis

Some people never experience any discernable symptoms of PUD and only find out they have ulcers when the disease causes a problem, such as bleeding or obstruction. The elderly and children are more likely to be the ones who do not report symptoms. The symptoms of gastric ulcers may be quite different from those of duodenal ulcers, which cause typical symptoms in only 50 percent of people.

The typical symptoms of duodenal ulcers include gnawing, burning, aching, an empty feeling, and hunger. An interesting aspect of duodenal ulcers is that eating tends to alleviate pain and other symptoms. For many years this confounded attempts to treat ulcers, falsely giving the impression that food could cause or cure the disease. In gastric ulcers, however, eating causes symptoms, sometimes even quite severe pain. The reason is that inflammation is more common with these ulcers, preventing food from moving through to the small intestine. The result is bloating, nausea, and even vomiting after eating.

When a person goes to the doctor complaining of stomach pain, PUD is top on the list of likely suspects. The tests for diagnosing PUD include endoscopy, blood tests, X rays with contrast, and analysis of stomach secretions (see Figure 4.4). Endoscopy allows the physician to see ulcers, although 5 to 10 percent of both types of ulcers will not be detected this way. The benefits of endoscopy are that a biopsy can be taken to find out if an ulcer is malignant and that it can stop bleeding.

An X ray with barium contrast is the same as the process for esophageal studies, but in this case, the stomach is of interest. Also called an upper GI, this test is helpful in finding ulcers that aren't

- Endoscopy

- Upper GI (barium swallow with X ray)

- Gastric analysis

- Blood tests to detect anemia (hemoglobin, hematocrit, mean-cell volume, and mean-cell hemoglobin), and *H. pylori*

Figure 4.4 Diagnostic Tests for Peptic Ulcer Disease

visible with endoscopy. The X ray, however, may not spot up to 20 percent of ulcers. Gastric analysis involves suctioning fluid from the stomach, which can provide information on the level of acid secretions. Usually, physicians use this method if the PUD is severe, if surgery will be performed, or if ulcers return after treatment. Blood tests can tell the physician if the person is infected with *H. pylori* or if anemia developed from bleeding ulcers.

Research Update on PUD

If British scientists have their way, the uncomfortable procedure of endoscopy will be a thing of the past. Researchers affiliated with the Royal London Hospital developed a wireless capsule endoscope, which they recently tested on ten patients. The mechanism, a swallowable electronic radiotelemetry capsule, is small enough (11 by 33 millimeters) to be swallowed rather easily. The procedure also does away with the need for the infusion of air, which is also uncomfortable, because the capsule is propelled along the length of the GI tract by peristalsis. After the capsule is swallowed, it sends video feedback by UHF-band radiotelemetry that can transmit continuously for over five hours. The capsule caused no discomfort among the patients and was easily expelled in about a day.[6] The procedure needs more testing before becoming available, and current endoscopy, although uncomfortable, still offers significant advantages. With the use of an endoscope, instruments can be attached and manipulated through the endoscope, allowing for tissue biopsy and treatment, such as to stop GI bleeding.

It is well known that fruits and vegetables are a great source of a variety of nutrients, but they may also decrease your risk of disease. Data from the 1993 Italian Household Multipurpose Survey, based on a sample of 46,693 subjects, analyzed the relationship between frequency of vegetable consumption and prevalence of twelve chronic diseases.[7] Many of the chronic diseases, including peptic ulcer disease, had an inverse relationship with vegetable consumption. Fruits and vegetables are rich sources of nutrients, including vitamins, trace minerals, and dietary fiber. They also contain many other active compounds, including phytochemicals. Phytochemicals work by a variety of mechanisms, including stimulation of the immune system, detoxification, modulating hormone metabolism, reducing blood pressure, reduction of platelet aggregation, and antiviral and antibacterial effects.[8]

Although there is no doubt eating a variety of fruits and vegetables every day is a good health practice, it is hard to determine whether the relationship between their consumption and decreased risk of disease is causal. Researchers have found that those who reported the lowest intake of fruits and vegetables were also more likely to report that they were sedentary, were heavy smokers, and were heavy drinkers.[9] Fruit and vegetable intake varies with several other chronic disease risk factors, which should be kept in mind when analyzing experimental studies.

Since the discovery of *H. pylori*, psychological factors have been discounted as a cause of peptic ulcer disease. There is solid evidence, however, that psychological stress triggers many ulcers and impairs response to treatment. In addition, most people infected with *H. pylori* do not develop ulcers, so the organism cannot serve as the sole explanation for ulcer disease.

Studies have found an excess of life stressors in ulcer patients compared with matched controls, but the effects of stress seem to be reversible. A person who develops an ulcer during a stressful period is likely to remain free of symptoms for years after a short course of treatment, even without medication to eradicate *H. pylori.*

Researchers think that psychological stress probably interacts with *H. pylori* and other risk factors in causing ulcers.[10] It may act by stimulating the production of gastric acid or by promoting behavior that causes a risk to health, such as smoking or taking nonsteroidal anti-inflammatory drugs. Although exact modes of action between stress, *H. pylori,* and other risk factors are only speculative, further research is warranted on the effects of psychosocial factors on peptic ulcer disease.

Approximately 13 million people in the United States regularly take nonsteroidal anti-inflammatory drugs (NSAIDs) for arthritis. Studies have shown, however, that 2 to 4 percent of patients who take an NSAID for a year develop serious gastrointestinal complications, including ulcers and bleeding from the stomach and small intestine. Colostrum, the milk a woman produces for the first few days after giving birth, is a rich natural source of nutrients, antibodies, and growth factors. It may be of value in eliminating infection and stimulating growth of the newborn infant's gastrointestinal tract. Its benefit in the prevention and treatment of adult gastrointestinal injury is now being explored.

A recent study examined whether spray-dried, defatted colostrum or milk preparations could prevent stomach and small intestinal injury induced by the NSAID indomethacin. The study used several well-validated test-tube and animal studies. The form of colostrum used in this experiment is commercially available as a health food supplement in the United States, the United Kingdom, and Europe. It is marketed as a general "health-promoting" product, particularly for athletes.

The results of the study showed that stomach and small intestinal injury caused by indomethacin could be reduced by colostrum and that a similarly prepared milk solution was far less effective. Colostrum caused a dose-dependent reduction in the amount of gastric injury. The cell studies used cells of both rats and humans to show that these effects were not species specific. The authors of this study concluded that bovine colostrum could provide a new approach for the prevention and treatment of the damaging effects of NSAIDs on the gut.[11] Further studies are under way to determine its value in patients taking long-term NSAIDs and in the treatment of other conditions of the bowel, where treatment is also suboptimal.

Evidence that the decline of peptic ulcer disease is attributable to the rising consumption of polyunsaturated fatty acids (PUFAs) has been accumulating. This decline may be due to the increase in synthesis of prostaglandins, which are protective of cells.[12] PUFAs are also known to inhibit the growth of H. pylori, which is the most likely cause for the development of ulcers.[13]

In one recent study, rats were induced with steroids to cause gastric ulceration and were fed PUFA supplements in the form of fish oil and arachidonic-rich oil.[14] The steroid-induced ulceration was associated with changes in the phospholipid fatty acid profile as well as other measures such as lipid peroxidation products, nitric oxide, and activity of antioxidant enzymes. PUFA supplementation decreased the incidence of ulceration, which was associated with normalizing the fatty acid profile. The other measures mentioned also reverted back to control values. The authors of the study concluded that this steroid-induced gastric ulceration was prevented by PUFAs.

Researchers now speculate that PUFAs could heal ulcers and protect the stomach lining.[15] More research is needed on humans before proposing fish oils or PUFA supplementation as treatment for ulcers, but as more evidence becomes available, PUFAs may be exploited as potential antipeptic ulcer agents.

Treatment and Nutritional Intervention

The history of PUD treatment is replete with regimens, some logical but ineffective, others potentially dangerous voodoolike therapies. Perhaps the most infamous is the Sippy diet, named for its physician-inventor Dr. Bertram W. Sippy in 1915. In its time, the Sippy diet was standard practice for many years, and variations on the theme persisted into recent history. The regimen consisted of a rigid program of milk and cream, progressing to soft foods, and presented as small, frequent meals. Because people with PUD who followed the regimen felt better, Sippy believed (and he was not alone) that milk had curative powers. The effect was probably because most people with PUD have duodenal ulcers and experience symptoms when their stomach is empty.

Rather than being curative, the Sippy diet may have been counterproductive in helping heal the ulcers; worse still, it was later associated with a high rate of coronary heart disease. This adverse side effect is not surprising considering the amount of saturated fat in full-fat dairy products, particularly heavy creams. As for the ulcers, milk actually increases acid secretion, as does eating frequency. Any time a person puts food into the stomach, digestive secretions, including acid, are stimulated.

The Sippy diet soon gave way to variations such as the bland diet, which was originally much stricter than its current form, and multi-stage ulcer diets that persisted into the 1980s at some facilities. The history of diet therapy in PUD illustrates beautifully the folly of using untested regimens. At the very least, regimens imposed needless dietary hardship, and at their worst, some lead to life-threatening complications, as in the case of the Sippy diet and associated heart disease.

Current treatment for PUD centers on determining the cause of the disease and, when it exists, eradicating *H. pylori* (see Figures 4.5 and 4.6). Although no conclusive evidence has shown that a bland diet affects the healing of ulcers, many people with PUD tend to prefer this type of diet, especially after a flare-up. The foods and substances to avoid are those that may irritate the mucosa or may increase acid secretion. Regarding acid, it's time to explode a perennial myth. Many people with ulcers believe that they should avoid acidic foods, such as tomatoes and citrus fruits, under the belief that these foods will cause or aggravate ulcers. Actually, eating any type of food tends to dilute the acidity of the stomach, because there isn't anything a person would normally eat that is more acidic than the acid level of the stomach. Even straight lemon and lime juice are both less acidic than stomach acid, so when these foods enter the stomach, they buffer the contents (lower the level of acid). Unless the ulcer sufferer is in the habit of ingesting car battery acid, there is no need to worry about the acid in food.

Objectives

1. Eradicate *H. pylori* infection if present.
2. Reduce gastric acidity and gastric secretion.
3. Avoid gastric irritants.
4. Promote ulcer healing.

Diet/Nutritional and Other Recommendations

1. Individualize the diet, or follow a bland diet if preferred.
2. Check for anemia (from bleeding ulcer); correct if present.
3. Check for B_{12} deficiency; correct if present.
4. Avoid large meals (they distend the stomach).
5. Avoid excessive alcohol.
6. Avoid caffeine and decaffeinated beverages.
7. Avoid cigarette smoking.
8. Include extra protein and vitamin C to promote healing.

Figure 4.5 Treatment Objectives and Dietary Recommendations for Peptic Ulcer Disease

Breakfast

- 1 banana
- 2 pieces of toast
- 2 teaspoons soybean margarine
- 1 cup 1 percent milk

Snack

- ⅔ cup Chex mix
- ½ cup fruit juice

Lunch

- 3 ounces tuna, packed in water
- 2 tablespoons low-calorie mayonnaise
- 2 slices whole-wheat bread
- 1 ounce pretzels
- 1 cup 1 percent milk
- 1 cup cantaloupe

Snack

- 1 cup low-fat cottage cheese
- 1 cup pineapple, juice packed, drained

Dinner

- 3 ounces broiled salmon
- ½ cup wild rice
- ½ cup boiled asparagus
- 1 cup 1 percent milk
- 1 cup strawberries
- 1 piece angel food cake
- 2 tablespoons whipped topping

Calories 2,065; protein 129 g (25%); fat 51 g (23%); carbohydrate 297 g (52%); cholesterol 162 mg; calcium 1,247 mg; sodium 3,200 mg; vitamin C 219 mg.

Figure 4.6 Sample Menu for Peptic Ulcer Disease and Gastritis

The subject of whether foods and other substances can irritate the intestinal mucosa is not clear. The traditional thinking was that substances such as red pepper and black pepper irritate and can potentially damage the mucosa. Over the years, however, several studies have yielded conflicting reports. Today, most experts agree that other than individualizing the diet, it may be best to be conservative and avoid potentially irritating substances. Some substances cause an increase in gastric secretion of acid and also are best avoided.

Smoking exerts many physiological effects on the stomach and duodenum, not the least of which are increased acid secretion and reduced acid-neutralizing bicarbonate from the pancreas. Because of these adverse effects, avoiding smoking is an important aspect of lifestyle change for treating PUD. Although this recommendation is standard, it has been challenged by research results that show no link between caffeine, alcohol, or smoking and duodenal ulcers.[16]

Other aspects of treatment include a variety of medications to accomplish the objectives of eradicating *H. pylori* if it is present, reducing acid secretion and gastric acidity, and promoting ulcer healing (see Figure 4.7). The H_2 antagonists and proton pump inhibitors (also called gastric acid pump inhibitors) inhibit acid secretion, although by different means. These drugs include cimetidine, famotidine, ranitidine, nizatidine, omeprazole, and lansoprazole. In contrast, other drugs such as sucralfate work by shoring up defenses. Sucralfate forms a protective gel that adheres to the ulcer site and prevents acid from penetrating and further damaging the mucosa. The drug misoprostol both inhibits acid secretion, especially during the night, and increases production of protective mucus.

Surgery Even when the underlying cause of PUD is *H. pylori,* experts estimate that 10 to 20 percent of cases will be difficult to treat. Treatment usually involves trying different antibiotics when previous drugs have failed. Even though treatment today is much more effective than

Antacids

Antibiotics (if H. pylori *present)*

Ulcer drugs
- H₂ antagonists (cimetidine/Tagamet, famotidine/Pepcid, nizatidine/ Axid, ranitidine/Zantac)
- omeprazole/Prilosec, lansoprazole/Prevacid
- sucralfate/Carafate
- misoprostol/Cytotec

Figure 4.7 Common Medications for Peptic Ulcer Disease

in the past, surgery is sometimes needed because of complications such as perforation, obstruction, or cancer.

The surgeries performed are partial (also called subtotal) or total gastrectomy (the removal of a portion or the entire stomach and duodenum) and vagotomy (cutting the nerve that senses pain and stimulates acid release). Even though surgery is necessary and sometimes prevents death, it also carries risks. Aside from the risk of the surgery itself, nutritional problems such as nutrient malabsorption, poor food intake, and weight loss can arise. Surgery can also cause a common disorder, dumping syndrome, that often leads to all these nutritional problems. A look at the surgeries sheds light on how dumping syndrome develops.

Common surgeries performed are the truncal vagotomy and pyloroplasty, the truncal vagotomy and antrectomy, and the highly selective vagotomy (see Figure 4.8). The truncal vagotomy is an aggressive surgery and can be of one of two types, the Billroth I (gastroduodenostomy) or the Billroth II (gastrojejunostomy) (see Figure 4.9). In the Billroth I procedure, the surgeon removes the lower portion of the stomach and then reattaches the remaining stomach to the duodenum. The Billroth II procedure involves removing up to 75 percent of

Truncal vagotomy and pyloroplasty

The truncal vagotomy cuts the main trunks of the vagus nerve on each side of the distal esophagus; it eliminates nerve-induced secretion of acid; it also reduces contractions and delays gastric emptying. To offset these effects, a pyloroplasty is also done. In the pyloroplasty, the pylorus is surgically altered so that it can act as a barrier to contents of the stomach as it empties. The result is that liquids empty more quickly, but solids take longer.

Truncal vagotomy and antrectomy

This procedure is more aggressive than truncal vagotomy and pyloroplasty, because the antrectomy connects the antrum and pylorus. When the antrum is altered, the portion of the stomach that secretes gastrin (the hormone that stimulates all gastric secretions) is removed. The two surgical procedures for attaching the remaining stomach to the intestine are called *Billroth I* and *Billroth II*.

Highly selective vagotomy (proximal gastric vagotomy)

This procedure reduces gastric acid secretion but does not interfere with motility—the stomach's movement—thus preventing problems related to gastric emptying, such as dumping syndrome.

Figure 4.8 Surgeries for Peptic Ulcer Disease

the stomach and the duodenum and reattaching the remaining stomach to the jejunem.

Surgery will likely affect all the major functions of the stomach to some extent, and the resulting problems depend on the surgery. The greater the amount of stomach tissue removed, the more severe and persistent the problems. The stomach's functions include serving as a reservoir for food, performing mechanical and enzymatic digestion, and producing of the intrinsic factor for vitamin B_{12} absorption.

The major nutritional complication, dumping syndrome, reflects the problems with these functions of the stomach after surgery. Dumping syndrome is a group of symptoms that result from rapid emptying of

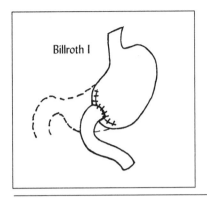
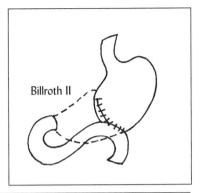

Figure 4.9 Surgeries for Peptic Ulcer

undigested food into the jejunum from the stomach. After stomach surgery, up to 50 percent of patients will have dumping syndrome, and the occurrence is extremely variable as to whom it affects and for how long. About 10 percent of patients who develop dumping syndrome have it for the rest of their lives. For most people, however, the stomach recovers after surgery and compensates for the loss in function.

Some people experience two different phases of dumping syndrome, early and late; others only have one phase; some have both. The early phase develops within twenty to ninety minutes after eating and consists of gastrointestinal and vasomotor symptoms. The gastrointestinal symptoms are typical of any digestive problem and include abdominal distention and pain, nausea, vomiting, and possibly diarrhea. The vasomotor symptoms are sweating, flushing, low blood pressure, a racing heartbeat, and dizziness.

The gastrointestinal symptoms start when the undigested contents of the stomach empty too quickly into the intestine, causing abdominal distention and pain; other symptoms follow. The vasomotor symptoms occur because as the undigested food enters the small intestine, fluid is pulled in from surrounding tissue to dilute the food. The fluid comes from blood vessels to enter the intestine, making blood pressure drop quickly and causing the vasomotor symptoms. Early dumping syndrome is a consequence of surgery that either reduced stomach capacity or removed a portion of the small intestine.

Late dumping occurs two to three hours after eating, with symptoms of dizziness, weakness, nausea, and sweating. The cause of late dumping is hypoglycemia, or low blood sugar. When carbohydrates in the food dump quickly into the small intestine, they are absorbed into the blood too quickly. The result is a spike in blood sugar, which in turn produces an oversecretion of insulin, driving blood sugar too low.

The treatment for dumping syndrome starts with a postgastrectomy diet or antidumping diet and may include drugs to slow gastric emptying (see Figures 4.10 and 4.11). The purposes of the diet are to control the symptoms of dumping syndrome and to prevent hypoglycemia. Foods containing protein and fat are emphasized because they are digested more slowly than carbohydrate. Also, carbohydrate tends to attract water into the intestine more rapidly than fat and protein. Another aspect of such a diet is small frequent meals to reduce the amount of food in the stomach and to help prevent hypoglycemia. The stomach contents can also be reduced by drinking liquids about one hour before or after a meal. Avoiding desserts and other sources of sugar may also help prevent hypoglycemia and rapid gastric emptying. Lying down after eating can help to slow movement of food from the stomach to the intestine. Because the small intestine produces the enzyme to digest lactose, lactose intolerance tends to be a common problem after surgery.

Other Nutritional Problems After Surgery Stomach surgery can cause problems with the absorption of iron because the lower acid level in the stomach does not favor the mineral's absorption. In addition, stomach surgery often bypasses the duodenum or food moves too quickly through it, and the duodenum is the main site of iron absorption. Poor food intake before surgery or bleeding ulcers also compromise iron status.

Foods to Avoid:
- Concentrated sweets (i.e., soft drinks, juices, pies, cakes, cookies, desserts made with sugar).
- Foods containing lactose (i.e., milk, milk products, cream soups, ice cream). Some aged cheeses and unsweetened yogurt may be tolerated.

Try to:
- Obtain 30 to 40 percent of calories from fat.
- Obtain 20 percent of calories from protein.
- Obtain 50 to 60 percent of calories from carbohydrates.
- Obtain 0 to 15 percent of calories from simple sugars.
- Consume 3 grams of sodium or less daily.
- Increase intake of fiber, especially pectin (found in fruits and vegetables, especially apples and citrus fruit).
- Use artificial sweeteners for beverages and desserts.

Dietary/Behavior Modifications:
- After surgery, avoid eating until the function of the gastrointestinal tract returns.
- Begin with sips of water at room temperature or allow ice chips to melt in mouth.
- Proceed to a clear liquid diet.
- When tolerated, begin a full liquid diet.
- As solids are introduced, begin with small amounts of soft, starchy, low-fat, low-protein foods.
- Eat small, frequent meals.
- Avoid large amounts of liquids with meals. Drink fluids one to two hours before or after meals.
- Avoid activity and lie down for one hour after meals.
- Avoid extremes in food temperature.

Possible Diet and Surgery-Induced Deficiencies:
- Iron
- Calcium
- Vitamin D
- Riboflavin
- Folacin
- Vitamin B_{12}

Figure 4.10 Postgastrectomy Dietary Recommendations

Breakfast

1   egg, scrambled
¾   cup oatmeal
1   tablespoon raisins
1   teaspoon margarine
      decaffeinated coffee (one hour after meal)

Snack

1   ounce dry-roasted almonds
1   apple

Lunch

3   ounces oven-roasted turkey breast
2   slices cracked-wheat bread
1   tablespoon low-calorie mayonnaise
1   medium carrot
1   cup blueberries
      iced tea (one hour after meal)

Snack

2   graham cracker squares
2   tablespoons crunchy peanut butter

Dinner

7.8   ounces pepper, stuffed with beef, rice, and tomato sauce
1   whole-wheat dinner roll
2   teaspoons margarine
1   cup steamed broccoli
1   pear
1   cup soy milk (one hour after meal)

Snack

2   ounces chicken salad
      rye crackers

Calories 1,880; protein 90 g (19%); fat 79 g (33%); carbohydrate 228 g
(48%); cholesterol 387 mg; calcium 604 mg; sodium 3,015 mg; fiber 25 mg.

Figure 4.11 Sample Postgastrectomy Menu

Another common problem after surgery for PUD is osteomalacia, or adult rickets. The cause of the disease is not clear, but it may be related to poor absorption of calcium. As with iron, the duodenum is an important absorption site for calcium. A contributing factor may be the chronic use of aluminum-containing antacids, which interfere with calcium and cause osteomalacia.

If the surgery was a total gastrectomy, a B_{12} supplement is warranted because the stomach cells produce the intrinsic factor for the vitamin's absorption. It is important to check vitamin B_{12} status because people taking a supplement of the B vitamin folate will be covering up symptoms of B_{12} deficiency.

Some gastric surgeries leave a section of the intestine bypassed, called *blind loop*, and peristalsis through that portion is cut off. This situation is similar to a stagnant pool of water, and bacteria can thrive and cause problems. Other ways gastric surgery can contribute to bacterial overgrowth is by reducing acid secretion, which normally helps keep bacteria in check, and by slowing peristalsis. Bacterial overgrowth can cause several nutritional problems, but the main concern is fat malabsorption. The bacteria damage bile, which is needed to emulsify fat for digestion, so fat cannot be broken down and absorbed. The energy from fat, which is more than twice that provided by carbohydrate and protein, is lost along with nutrients that require fat for absorption, such as vitamins A, D, E, and K. When fat is not absorbed by the small intestine, it passes to the colon, causing a type of fat-containing diarrhea called steatorrhea. To make matters worse, the bacteria compete with the person for vitamin B_{12} and folate. If the person finds it difficult to replace the energy and nutrients lost, weight loss and malnutrition often result. Treatment consists of antibiotics to stop bacterial growth and dietary measures including a low-fat diet, replacement of lost energy, and fat-soluble nutrients. If these measures fail, another surgery may be necessary to repair the loop.

Part III

Diseases of the Lower Gastrointestinal Tract

■ · · · · · · ■

I stood quietly at the doorway of Kathy's hospital room, observing as two of my students interviewed the young pregnant woman, clearly embarrassed at having to ask questions about her bowel regularity. With the diagnosis of ulcerative colitis and the often severe symptoms and life-threatening complications that attend it, Kathy's pregnancy could be in jeopardy. Because the disease can deplete nutrient levels, it was important to conduct a thorough assessment of her nutritional status. Kathy shifted beneath the stiff white sheets, in obvious physical discomfort, maybe because of some on-again, off-again, sharp abdominal pain or maybe because of the IV needle in her forearm that she tried unsuccessfully not to fiddle with.

Kathy also looked like she could use a diversion from the sterile gray walls and white-coated workers sporting beguiling little baskets in the crook of their arms, little baskets that upon closer inspection contained gruesome blood-filled tubes, looking to do a bit more blood-letting. At times, my two students would inadvertently provide a comedic distraction. When one finally stammered out the delicate question, "Do you have any bowel habits?" Kathy couldn't do anything but laugh.

Although the student's question was funny, there is nothing amusing about inflammatory bowel disease (IBD), especially about what happens during a flare-up. Some people with IBD may experience severe pain and twenty or more bowel movements a day, sometimes consisting of bloody diarrhea, when the disease is active. The two types of IBD, Crohn's disease and colitis, share several similar features, but tend to distinguish themselves eventually. In Kathy's case, the admitting diagnosis was "exacerbation [flare-up] of ulcerative colitis," which was not surprising because she had been diagnosed as a young teenager. In the interview, she had told the students that it took doctors a long time to figure out what was wrong with her.

One of the students ran up to me the next day, excited as only a first-time dietetics student could be at the news. "They changed her diagnosis!" she said. "They said she doesn't have colitis. She has Crohn's disease." That switch in diagnosis shows how difficult it can be to figure out which disease a person has. Although the news was interesting from an academic view, it was not good news for Kathy. Both diseases can be devastating to a person's health and quality of life, but because of where Crohn's disease strikes and does its damage, her first diagnosis would have been better. A strange fact about Crohn's disease is that pregnancy can cause a worsening or an improvement of the disease, with a fifty–fifty chance of either outcome.

This section reviews diseases of the lower GI tract, which includes the small intestine and large intestine, or colon. The various diseases often produce similar symptoms, such as diarrhea, constipation, and flatulence. The problems are generally rooted in a glitch in the mechanics of the lower GI tract: secretions, motility, digestion, and absorption in the small intestine, and reabsorption in the colon.

CHAPTER 5

Diarrhea, Lactose Intolerance, and Constipation

■ · · · · · · ■

DIARRHEA

Diarrhea is a Greek word that means "to flow through," and that describes diarrhea fairly well. It is a symptom, not a disease, and a common symptom of many lower GI diseases. Defining diarrhea can be a bit tricky, because normal bowel movement frequency and stool consistency can differ from one person to another. The best example of this variability is one used by a renowned nutrition researcher when speaking on the topic of fiber. Dr. David Jenkins, on discussing the study of dietary fiber in Africa, reports that because fiber intake is so high, subjects can often produce a stool sample for researchers on demand. Recognizing this individual variation, diarrhea is considered a change from usual bowel habits to those of higher fluid content, and it is often associated with increased frequency.

The problem with diarrhea, aside from the extremely unpleasant condition itself, are the serious metabolic consequences it brings about (see Table 5.1). The metabolic consequences can prove fatal in short order if they continue unchecked. Diarrhea is one of the leading causes of death among infants and young children worldwide. For most Americans, diarrhea is a self-limiting condition brought on by either viral or bacterial infection. In fact, one of the most common causes is food poisoning. For

Table 5.1 Consequences of Diarrhea

Excess Loss of . . .	Consequence
Fluid	Dehydration
Sodium	Hyponatremia
Potassium	Hypokalemia
Bicarbonate	Acidosis

some people, however, diarrhea is a symptom of a chronic disease affecting the lower GI, such as ulcerative colitis or Crohn's disease.

Because of its potentially life-threatening consequences, it is important to know how to treat diarrhea, which means understanding its different types (see Table 5.2). Osmotic diarrhea is caused by a compound entering the intestine that cannot be absorbed. The intestine's inability to absorb it may be because the intestine lacks enough of the enzyme needed to break down the compound. For example, with lactose intolerance, a person does not have enough lactase, the enzyme to break down lactose, so the compound cannot be absorbed in the small intestine. Instead, it moves intact into the colon, where it produces several effects that cause diarrhea.

The first effect of a lactose deficiency is similar to what occurs in the small intestine during dumping syndrome (see chapter 4), and it is the same type of diarrhea that the syndrome causes. Fluid floods into the colon from surrounding tissue in a process called an osmotic shift. Osmosis dictates that fluid will move across a membrane from the side with a higher concentration to the side with the lower concentration. Because the compound was not broken down and remained intact, it had this osmotic power; such a compound is called an *osmotically active particle*. Besides enzyme deficiencies leaving a compound intact, other substances act as osmotically active particles. Examples of other such

Table 5.2 Classification of Diarrhea

Type	Cause
Osmotic	Osmotically active particles
Secretory	Disease-induced H_2O secretion into intestinal lumen
Change in motility, transit time	Problem with hypermotility of GI tract
Iatrogenic	Caused by treatment, such as medications

compounds are certain laxatives, such as Milk of Magnesia. In this case, the presence of mineral salts in the colon produces the effect.

The second effect of a lactase deficiency is that bacteria that live in the colon do have enough of the enzyme to break down the lactose. They do so and in the process of fermentation cause the release of gases and acid. The higher level of acid produces a cathartic effect, adding to the problem of diarrhea. A significant fact about osmotic diarrhea is that fasting usually relieves this type of diarrhea.

A second type of diarrhea is secretory diarrhea, which is caused by disease processes that result in high secretions of water into the intestine. Secretory diarrhea can be a consequence of a disease that causes high pressure in the GI tract, usually either inflammation or obstruction. Another way it can occur is if something stimulates a specific cellular enzyme system. The most common trigger is a toxin produced by bacteria, either those that normally inhabit the colon or those present in contaminated food. Another trigger is bile salts, which are normally absorbed in the last segment of the small intestine but which end up in the colon. Diseases such as Crohn's disease and celiac disease, however, may affect that portion of the small intestine and hinder its ability to reabsorb bile salts. Secretory diarrhea causes much higher losses of fluid than does osmotic diarrhea, so dehydration is a great concern. In addition, fasting does not relieve secretory diarrhea.

Changes in muscle tone of the GI tract will change motility and transit time, resulting in the type of diarrhea that occurs in irritable bowel syndrome (see chapter 6). Some medications can produce iatrogenic diarrhea, so named to indicate that a treatment is causing the problem. With iatrogenic diarrhea, it is important to weigh the advantages of the treatment against the side effect. Sometimes, the body can adjust to the medication, and the diarrhea will resolve. Yet because of the potential for malnutrition with chronic diarrhea, it is important to monitor carefully the frequency of diarrhea and possible deficits in nutritional status.

Intestinal Gas and Flatulence

Gassiness, or flatulence, often accompanies diarrhea, although it can be a problem in its own right for many people. Although the subject of countless off-color jokes, it is not funny for people who have chronic gas. Gas is normally present in the GI tract as nitrogen, oxygen, carbon dioxide, hydrogen, and methane, and most people excrete about 700 milliliters of gas each day.[1] The sources of gas in the GI tract include swallowing air, chemical reactions in the colon, and exchange of gas between the bloodstream and the GI tract. The body has two ways of ridding itself of gas: by belching and by passing it rectally. A certain amount of gas excretion is normal, but an excessive amount, which is the definition of flatulence, can indicate the presence of disease. Most gases are reabsorbed in the colon as the feces moves through the organ; if the feces moves too quickly, as with diarrhea, there is not enough time for reabsorption and flatulence results.

Aerophagia, or swallowing air, causes belching; the gases involved are nitrogen and oxygen. Although not much swallowed air can reach the colon, when nitrogen and oxygen are high in rectal gas the cause is aerophagia. Normally, rectal gas is not analyzed, but if it were, it would make determining its cause easier. The treatment for aerophagia is to eat more slowly, chew with the mouth closed (always a good idea), and avoid drinking through straws.

The presence of hydrogen, carbon dioxide, and sometimes methane indicates that the culprit is bacterial fermentation. Such fermentation occurs most often when a person is not digesting and absorbing a carbohydrate in the small intestine and the intact compound is therefore entering the colon. In the colon, bacteria act on the carbohydrate, and one by-product is gas. After ruling out a malabsorption problem, such as lactose intolerance, a thorough look at the diet can help identify foods that are providing the fodder for the microbes. The most notorious abettors are the legumes, because they contain two indigestible carbohydrates, stachyose and raffinose. Conventional wisdom has been that eating legumes more frequently can lead to better tolerance, and legumes provide such nutrition and health benefits that it is worth the attempt.

A high-fiber diet in general produces flatulence in most people, especially if that diet is a new regimen. Any dietary change should be approached gradually, and increased fiber is no exception. Individually, several other foods such as cruciferous vegetables are gas-formers. These vegetables, such as broccoli, kale, and cabbage, smell like rotten eggs, which is attributable to the sulfur they contain. Cruciferous vegetables do produce this odor when cooked, so when eaten raw they do not have the same effect for most people. Some people have flatulence after eating certain fruits, such as apples, raisins, and cantaloupe, but there is much individual variation in response to these foods. Two food additives, sorbitol (an artificial sweetener) and fructose (a natural sweetener), can also cause gas problems, but it is generally the overuse of these sweeteners that causes the problem. The commercial product Bean-O can be useful for some people; it can be added to cooked foods or taken orally to help prevent gas.

Flatulence may be a sign of GI malabsorption or disease that could become serious if not diagnosed and treated and thus should be checked out by a physician. After disease has been ruled out, the most useful approach is a careful assessment of diet habits and the trial-and-error process of adding and omitting certain foods.

Treatment

Diarrhea in infants and young children and in the elderly is a special concern. These groups are at a higher risk for dehydration, which is the major short-term concern of diarrhea. In fact, dehydration is a common hospital admitting diagnosis for an elderly person. If diarrhea is chronic and does not respond to treatment, it is called intractable diarrhea, which is a serious condition. Thus, it is critical to stay on top of the situation, watching for any signs of dehydration or, longer term, malnutrition and seeking medical attention quickly. If diarrhea lasts one to four days and is not accompanied by vomiting, it can be treated at home (see Figures 5.1 and 5.2). Several medications can help relieve persistent diarrhea. If a bug is causing the diarrhea, however, it is best to let the infection work its way through the GI tract. Antidiarrheal medications slow the GI tract, keeping the toxin in the system longer and maintaining the infection.

LACTOSE INTOLERANCE

Some experts have said that because lactose intolerance (LI; also lactose malabsorption or lactase deficiency) is so common, affecting up to 75 percent of the world's population, that it should be considered the normal state. LI occurs in 70 percent of Africans, 95 percent of Asians, and 10 percent of Americans and Hispanics, although

Treatment
- Eliminate or control underlying disease.
- Correct fluid and mineral imbalances.
- Medications.
- No food, only clear liquids.

For diarrhea lasting only up to four days (without vomiting)
- Withhold foods for twenty-four hours.
- Push clear fluids, especially fruit juices (not milk).
- In infants, use rehydration solution, such as Pedialyte.
- Progress to a low-fiber diet before returning to a regular diet.

Medications to Relieve Diarrhea
- Atropine sulfate
- Bismuth subsalicylate
- Diphenoxylate
- Kaolin- and pectin-containing drugs
- Loperamide
- Tincture of opium

Figure 5.1 Treating Diarrhea

researchers have suggested that it is overdiagnosed. The three types of LI are congenital, primary or genetic, and secondary or acquired. Congenital LI is rare and is present at birth. In primary LI, which is uncommon among children but common in adults, the GI cells do not make sufficient levels of lactase. Secondary LI is a result of another disease process that affects the GI tract. Two examples are Crohn's disease and celiac disease, which both affect the small intestine. As the intestinal cells become damaged, they are no longer able to produce the enzymes, such as lactase, that they normally make.

As discussed previously, lactose enters the colon intact and produces GI symptoms by several means. The symptoms of LI include

Breakfast

¾   cup oatmeal

1   slice white toast

1   teaspoon margarine
    decaffeinated tea

8   ounces Ensure

Snack

½   cup applesauce

2   graham cracker squares

Lunch

12   ounces high-protein beef broth

6   saltines

½   cup mashed potatoes

1   banana
    decaffeinated tea

Dinner

12   ounces high-protein chicken broth

½   cup chicken-flavored rice

½   cup fruit cocktail (in juice)

8   ounces Ensure

Snack

5   ounces high-protein gelatin

Calories 2,040; protein 81 g (16%); fat 38 g (17%); carbohydrate 335 g (70%); cholesterol 22 mg; calcium 548 mg; sodium 3,671 mg.

Figure 5.2a Sample Menu for Diarrhea in Acute Stage

Breakfast
1	cup fruit yogurt
2	slices French toast
1	teaspoon margarine
1	ounce syrup
	decaffeinated coffee

Snack
½	cup mandarin oranges (in juice)
10	animal crackers

Lunch
8	ounces macaroni and cheese
½	cup green beans
1	cup 1 percent milk
1	cup watermelon

Snack
1	slice banana bread

Dinner
3	ounces meat loaf
½	cup mashed sweet potatoes
½	cup sliced beets
1	kiwi fruit

Snack
1	ounce pretzels

Calories 2,038; protein 74 g (15%); fat 59 g (26%); carbohydrate 297 g (59%); cholesterol 319 mg; calcium 1,156 mg; sodium 3,336 mg.

Figure 5.2b Sample Menu for Diarrhea in Acute Stage as Tolerance Improves

bloating, cramping, nausea, flatulence (gassiness), and diarrhea. Lactose enters into the GI tract as a carbohydrate contained in mainly dairy products and makes up about 10 percent of the total carbohydrate in the average American diet (see Table 5.3). Although dairy products contain the most lactose, there are some exceptions. Yogurt contains the same amount of lactose as milk, but most types also contain lactase to break it down and are better tolerated than milk. Natural cheeses usually contain only small amounts of lactose, but processed cheese food slices contain a bit more because of added milk solids. Because manufacturers often use the dairy food component whey as a filler ingredient in other foods, it is important to read ingredient labels. In addition, lactose itself is sometimes used as a filler in medications, such as Maalox, Premarin, and Contact.

Research Update on Lactose Intolerance

Some people may be avoiding dairy products because of a perceived intolerance to lactose. For example, calcium intakes of female African-American adolescents are approximately 730 milligrams per day, whereas the adequate intake for adolescents is 1,300 milligrams. Several studies have reported that people with lactose maldigestion develop improved tolerance to lactose following repeated exposure to dairy foods containing lactose. The mechanism for this adaptation is likely an alteration in the metabolic activity of the colon's microflora.

A recent study determined whether African-American adolescent girls who were fed a dairy-rich diet could adapt to lactose.[2] The subjects consumed a dairy-based diet averaging 1,200 milligrams of calcium and 33 grams of lactose per day for twenty-one days. Lactose digestion was assessed by comparing breath hydrogen production (a measure of lactose maldigestion) and gastrointestinal symptoms at the beginning and at the end of the study. The results showed a sig-

Table 5.3 Lactose Content of Foods

Food	Serving Size	Lactose (grams)
Milk	1 cup	
whole		11
1 and 2 percent		9–13
skimmed		12–14
evaporated		24
sweetened, condensed		30
chocolate		10–12
buttermilk		9–11
lactase-treated		< 3
Cheese, processed	1 oz.	0.5–2.0
Cheese, natural	1 oz.	0.4–0.8
Cottage cheese	1 cup	5–8
Ice cream, ice milk	1 cup	9–10
Light cream	1 tbsp.	0.5
Sherbet	1 cup	4
Sour cream	1 tbsp.	< 1
Whipped topping	1 tbsp.	0.5
Yogurt	1 cup	11–15
Whey	variable (used as filler)	

nificant decrease in the amount of hydrogen produced on day twenty-one compared with day one. Gastrointestinal symptoms were negligible throughout the whole study, but there was a significant decrease in the severity of bloating and flatulence after adaptation to the diet. The authors concluded that the diet was well tolerated, and the decrease in breath hydrogen suggests colonic adaptation to the high-lactose diet. Therefore, lactose maldigestion should not be a restricting factor in developing adequate calcium diets. The study declared that dietetic practitioners can advise lactose-intolerant clients to include dairy foods with meals at levels that result in sufficient calcium to meet the recommended dietary intakes. Every case is different and some individuals can tolerate lactose better than others, but by consuming lactose with meals in moderate amounts throughout the day, LI should not be a limiting factor in obtaining adequate calcium.

Lactose maldigestion is the inability to completely digest lactose, the major carbohydrate found in milk. People with lactose maldigestion may experience abdominal pain, bloating, flatulence, and acute diarrhea.[3] A study in Sicily analyzed the relationship between lactose maldigestion, self-reported milk intolerance, and gastrointestinal symptoms in a randomized sample of 323 subjects.[4] Each participant's diet was investigated for seven consecutive days under the supervision of a team of dietitians. The subjects were then divided into self-reported milk-intolerants and self-reported milk-tolerants. They underwent hydrogen breath testing after a lactose load to determine those who were maldigesters. Those with one or more symptoms were classified as intolerants. The study found that the occurrence of lactose intolerance is much lower than that of lactose maldigestion. Of this population, 32 percent were lactose maldigesters but tolerants, whereas only 4 percent were lactose maldigesters and intolerants. Of those who reported themselves as milk intolerant, only 10 percent were lactose maldigesters and intolerants, and, surprisingly, 37 percent had no problem with lactose at all. Gastrointestinal symptoms were found in very few self-reported milk-intolerants. The entire group of self-reported milk-intolerants consumed significantly less milk and had lower calcium intakes than all the other subjects studied (320 milligrams/day versus 585 milligrams/day). The entire study group was significantly below the recommended intake level, however.

Many cases of self-diagnosed lactose intolerance are questionable.[5] In one controlled study, people claiming to have lactose intolerance were given cow's milk without knowing it, and the majority did not show any symptoms. When those same people were given lactose-reduced milk but were told it was regular cow's milk, many experienced stomach upsets.[6]

These studies have shown that many people who think that they are lactose intolerant may in fact be only maldigesters with negligible symptoms or may have no difficulty at all with the digestion of lactose. Therefore, many of these people may unnecessarily reduce their milk product consumption.

Researchers have reported that many lactose maldigesters tolerate more lactose in studies than in everyday life.[7] This finding has led to the possibility that symptoms of intolerance may be related to other carbohydrates as well. In a randomized, double-blind crossover study, forty women were classified into three groups: lactose maldigesters, control lactose digesters, and lactose digesters who report milk to be the cause of their gastrointestinal symptoms (pseudohypolactasic subjects). At different time intervals, the participants were given either 50 grams of lactose, 50 grams of sucrose, 25 grams of lactulose, or 25 grams of fructooligosaccharides. The last two carbohydrates were employed because they are classified as indigestible. Commonly used diagnostic methods for lactose maldigestion were used and compared.

The groups showed no significant difference in hydrogen production (a measure of lactose maldigestion) after ingesting sucrose and fructooligosaccharides.[8] Lactose maldigesters produced significantly more hydrogen after ingesting lactose and lactulose. Compared with the controls, symptoms were increased in the pseudohypolactasic subjects after ingestion of lactulose and fructooligosaccharides. All four carbohydrates increased symptoms in the lactose maldigesters. These results may explain the discrepancies between claims of lactose maldigestion and the results of studies. Both groups may be misinterpreting the cause of their symptoms. The symptoms of lactose maldigesters and pseudohypolactasic subjects may be caused by the ingestion of carbohydrates other than lactose.

Treatment

Treatment for LI consists of avoiding lactose (see Figure 5.3), using special products that digest lactose, or buying food in which the lactose is predigested. The special products such as Lact-Aid come in pill or drop form and can either be added to foods or taken prior to eating lactose-containing food. Most people with LI can tolerate 4 ounces of milk, one of the foods containing the most lactose, at one time. Tolerance is highly individual, however. Some people with LI experience severe symptoms even with small amounts of milk as an ingredient in another food item.

One way to increase tolerance of milk is to include it as part of a meal with other foods. Researchers have also reported that people with LI can increase their tolerance to lactose-containing foods by including small amounts each day and gradually increasing the amount over time. Dairy products are the best sources of calcium, in a form that the body absorbs best. People who avoid dairy products may need to consider a calcium supplement.

CONSTIPATION

As with diarrhea, a definition for constipation is somewhat difficult because of individual variation in what a person considers normal frequency. Many people feel constipated if they do not have a bowel movement each day, whereas others only consider one week to be the start of a problem. As a diagnosis, constipation exists when a per-

Breakfast
1   fried egg
1   slice toast
1   teaspoon soy margarine
1   tablespoon jam
1   cup calcium-fortified orange juice

Snack
1   cup calcium-fortified dry cereal

Lunch
3   slices ham
2   slices rye bread
1   teaspoon soy margarine
½   cup baked beans
1   orange
½   cup whole milk (if tolerated)

Dinner
8   ounces spaghetti with meat sauce
1   tablespoon grated Parmesan cheese (if tolerated)
1   piece corn bread
2   cups romaine salad
2   tablespoons vinegar and oil dressing
½   cup broccoli
1   cup calcium-fortified juice
½   cup honeydew melon

Snack
1   ounce dry-roasted almonds

Calories 2,070; protein 71 g (15%); fat 71 g (30%); carbohydrate 284 g (55%); cholesterol 306 mg; calcium 1,567 mg; sodium 4,678 mg.

Figure 5.3 Sample Menu for Lactose Intolerance

son eating a high-fiber diet has fewer than three bowel movements in one week or skips three days between movements. People with constipation experience a range of symptoms, including headache, anorexia, abdominal discomfort, lower back pain, and bloating. A short bout of constipation is normal and is probably the result of a change in dietary or lifestyle habits. Chronic constipation, however, is not something to take lightly, because the cause may be a serious condition such as a metabolic disorder or colon cancer. A quick review of how the system normally works helps describe problems that lead to constipation.

After a person eats a meal in the morning, the residue generally reaches the colon by the following morning. Peristalsis keeps the residue moving, albeit at the rather slow average speed of two inches per hour. The person will probably have a bowel movement that morning or up to forty-eight hours later. Many factors determine transit time, the time it takes for the residue of a meal to be excreted. Diet, especially the amount and type of fiber and the amount of fluid a person consumes, plays a major role. Other key influences are physical activity, being in an upright position to assist peristalsis, regularity in bowel habits, and attention to a special signal.

This special signal is the defecation reflex, and it sounds the alarm when the fecal mass, or stool, moves from the sigmoid colon to the rectum. As the fecal mass fills the rectum, it stretches and sets off nerve impulses in the lower portion of the spine, effecting the defecation reflex. The reflex is under voluntary control, so a person can ignore the urge if it is not convenient (a user-friendly design!). Each time the reflex is ignored, however, the stool moves back to the sigmoid colon. In this part of the colon, the colonic mucosa do what they are supposed to do with waste: reabsorb water. As water is reabsorbed, the stool becomes drier and harder, making it much more difficult to pass with the opportunity of the next reflex.

Ignoring the reflex is rather common in today's fast-paced lifestyle, but it is likely that such behavior, along with irregular bowel habits, is a major contributor to constipation. Besides diet and physical activity, there can be many other causes of constipation (see Figure 5.4). Diet, physical activity, and all these possible causes should be assessed when seeking an effective treatment for chronic constipation. Socioeconomic issues can be critical for some people with chronic constipation. If a large family has a small living space, with only one bathroom, it can be difficult for each person to establish regular bowel habits.

Decreased expulsive power and deficient peristaltic activity can be the result of aging, medications, a disease process that affects the nervous system or muscles, or some unknown cause. An obstruction that prevents movement of the stool through the colon can be caused by a tumor, by active inflammation from disease, or by impacted feces. People with psychologic problems (psychogenic) may have chronic constipation, and the cause is often multifactorial. Problems in metabolism and mineral disturbances, such as hypothyroidism and hypercalcemia, can also affect normal bowel movements. All these cases underscore the importance of seeing a physician to diagnose serious conditions.

- Low socioeconomic status
- Decreased expulsive power
- Deficient peristaltic activity
- Obstruction of movement
- Metabolic/mineral disorder
- Psychogenic issues

Figure 5.4 Causes of Constipation

Treatment

After a careful assessment of all the possible contributing factors of constipation, treatment can be more targeted. If disease processes are not causing the chronic constipation, the first measures are always diet, physical activity, and establishment of regular bowel habits, most notably, heeding the reflex. Most people think that they get enough fiber in their diet, but an actual analysis of their food intake would probably surprise them. Several health agencies recommend 20 to 35 grams of fiber each day, and this recommendation is for someone who is not having constipation problems. Middle-aged and older women who are less active and need fewer calories (about 1,600) per day are at the lower end of the fiber range, and teenaged boys and active men are at the higher end. To achieve this recommendation, a major part of the diet would have to consist of fruits, vegetables, and whole grains (see Table 5.4). Most Americans do not come close to these recommendations. Those trying to increase fiber intake should do so gradually; they will probably have GI discomfort, especially cramping and gassiness, on a high-fiber diet.

Adequate fluid intake is just as important as fiber. Fiber helps to promote good bowel health by acting like a sponge to attract water into the stool. The stool swells and gently pushes against the muscle wall of the colon, encouraging peristalsis and softening so that the stool is easier to pass. Constipation can actually be aggravated if someone increases fiber intake but has poor fluid intake. The fluid need of the average person is 1 milliliter for every calorie consumed (see Table 5.5). If someone is extremely active, engaging in thiry minutes of strenuous aerobic activity more than three times each week, he or she needs to replace all that sweat with more fluid. In addition, people who work outdoors at strenuous labors, especially in a hot climate, will need more fluid than the average person.

Table 5.4 Fiber Content of Foods

Food	Serving Size	Fiber (grams)
Bread and cereal		
whole wheat	1 slice	2
cereal, bran	1 ounce	2
cooked oatmeal	½ cup	2
Fruit		
apple, banana, kiwi, pear	1 medium	2
Legumes		
baked beans, kidney beans, navy beans	½ cup	8
garbanzo, lima beans, lentils, split peas	½ cup	5
Vegetables		
cooked broccoli, cooked corn, cooked green beans, cooked winter squash	½ cup	3
raw carrots, raw peppers	½ cup	3

Cathartics, popularly called *laxatives*, should not be the first step in a constipation treatment plan because they may cause side effects (see Table 5.6). Any laxative use should be only occasional because adverse side effects are more likely to arise with continual use. The less serious side effects include abdominal distention, nausea, cramping, and gassiness. More serious effects include malabsorption and diarrhea, reduced absorption of fat-soluble vitamins, interference with absorption of essential minerals, and imbalances of mineral blood levels. Figures 5.5 and 5.6 give guidance in dealing with constipation.

Table 5.5 Energy and Fluid Needs

Age/Gender Group	Energy (calories)	Fluid (cups)
Women, some older adults	1,600	6.7
Children, teenaged girls, active women, most men	2,200	9.2
Teenaged boys, active men	2,800	11.7

Not surprisingly, the cathartics most likely to cause these side effects are the more potent stimulant and saline cathartics, sometimes called *purgatives* and *drastics*. The stimulant cathartics are substances that irritate the GI tract, which increases motility. Examples are castor oil and the active ingredient in prune juice, phenolphthalein, which is the active ingredient in several commerical laxatives. The major problems with the overuse of phenolphthalein are depletion of potassium in the blood and reduced absorption of vitamin D, calcium, and other minerals. Saline laxatives are salts that the GI tract cannot absorb, so they move into the colon and produce diarrhea by an osmotic fluid shift. The major problem with these laxatives is their potential to bind essential minerals, such as calcium, and prevent their absorption. In

Table 5.6 Types of Cathartics

Cathartic Agent	Action
Emollient	Stool softeners, help water to penetrate stool
Bulk-forming	Fiber-containing, attracts water
Stimulant	Contain compounds that irritate GI tract
Saline	Mineral compounds that cause osmotic diarrhea because they are not absorbed

Figure 5.5 Dietary Recommendations for Constipation

- Fiber intake should be increased. (Exception: In spastic constipation, fiber intake should be decreased during painful episodes and then gradually increased.)

- Consume five to eight servings of fruits and vegetables daily (especially those with edible skins, seeds, and hulls).

- Consume six or more servings of whole-grain breads and cereals daily.

- Consume 25 grams of soluble and insoluble fiber daily in a 3:1 ratio.

  Soluble fiber sources: Apples, barley, carrots, citrus fruits, guar, legumes, oats, and strawberries.

  Insoluble fiber sources: Bran, fruits and edible seeds, vegetables, wheat, whole grains, whole-wheat flour.

  Other fiber sources: Prune juice, dried fruits, and nuts.

- Increase fluid intake to 8 to 10 cups daily, based on energy needs and calorie intake (warm fluids may be especially helpful).

- Increase fiber intake gradually to avoid painful gas and bloating. (Do not use excessive bran due to possible wheat allergy.)

- Exercise regularly.

- Do not ignore the need for a bowel movement; establish a routine for bowel habits.

Possible Modified Diet-Induced Deficiencies:
- Calcium

- Copper

- Iron

- Zinc

Figure 5.6 Sample Menu for Constipation

Breakfast

¾   cup bran flakes

1   cup 1 percent milk

½   cup raspberries

1   cup orange juice

Snack

1   pear

Lunch

2   slices cracked-wheat bread

2   tablespoons crunchy peanut butter

1   tablespoon jam

2   cups garden salad

2   tablespoons ranch dressing

1   apple

1   cup 1 percent milk

Snack

1   granola bar

½   cup pineapple

Dinner

3½   ounces broiled pork loin chop

1   medium baked potato with skin

2   teaspoons margarine

½   cup peas

3   medium apricots

1   cup 1 percent milk

Calories 2,053; protein 90 g (18%); fat 47 g (26%); carbohydrate 326 g (56%); cholesterol 108 mg; calcium 1,197 mg; sodium 1,301 mg; fiber 25 mg.

addition, they may act too dramatically and cause diarrhea, not a normal bowel movement.

Emollient, or stool-softeners, and bulk-forming laxatives are less powerful than salines and stimulants. Emollients work by helping water penetrate the stool, making it softer and easier to pass. The major side effects of emollients are nausea, anorexia, and diarrhea. Bulk-forming laxatives contain fiber, and fiber increases stool mass by attracting water. These laxatives can cause gas, and if taken chronically, they can also cause mineral imbalances. Even these more gentle laxatives should only be used occasionally. Aside from the serious side effects, laxative abuse can actually contribute to chronic constipation by interfering with the normal defecation reflex.

CHAPTER 6

Diverticular Disease and Irritable Bowel Syndrome

■ · · · · · · · ■

DIVERTICULOSIS AND DIVERTICULITIS

Diverticular disease is the presence of small outpockets, or herniations, of the colon, most often in the sigmoid colon (see Figure 6.1). Each pouch is called a diverticulum. Diverticula range in size from one-tenth of an inch to more than an inch, although the smaller size is more typical. The condition of having the pouches is the disease diverticulosis, and when the pouches become inflamed, the flare-up is diverticulitis. This condition is common in developed countries; experts estimate that 30 to 40 percent of Americans over the age of fifty have diverticulosis. The number is much higher as people move past the age of fifty. If a person makes it to age ninety, there is not much chance that he or she will not have diverticulosis. Thus, as the American population continues to grow older, more people will develop the disease.

Most people who have diverticulosis have no symptoms and are unaware that they have the disease until a diverticulum becomes inflamed and infected, sending them to the emergency room. Some experts now believe, however, that people with diverticulosis do have mild symptoms. The lack of noticeable symptoms makes it difficult to determine exactly how many people are affected. When a diverticulum

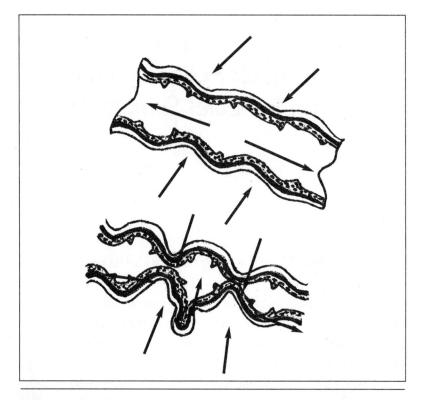

Figure 6.1 Theorized mechanism by which low-fiber diets promote diverticula. With bulky colon contents (*top*), muscle contractions exert pressure longitudinally. If the lumen is smaller (*bottom*), contractions can produce occlusion and exert pressure against the colon wall, which may produce a diverticular "blow-out"

first forms, it can easily disappear when pressure inside the colon falls, so the number of diverticula at any one time can vary. Eventually, however, the pouches cannot be reduced and become permanent fixtures with the walls of the colon. As stool moves through the colon on its way to the rectum, tiny amounts can enter the pouches. If it's early in the diverticulum's development and the diverticulum can be reduced, the feces is expelled as the pouch shrinks. If, however, the pouch has become permanent, the feces inside becomes thickened and stonelike, causing inflammation and infection, the condition of diverticulitis.

Serious complications can occur in diverticulitis, some of which are life threatening. For example, a diverticulum can rupture, causing bleeding and spreading infection throughout the body. The diverticulum can also cause an obstruction, blocking the flow of stool to the rectum. Although the mechanics of the causes of a flare-up are well understood, the cause of diverticulosis is still the subject of conjecture. The best theory suggests that diverticulosis is caused by a combination of high pressure inside the colon and a weakening in the organ's musculature. As to factors that can affect these two aspects of the colon's health, the answer is even more theoretical. Some factors that may act on either pressure (intracolonic pressure) or musculature are emotional stress, constipation, especially with straining, and GI motility and transit time. From a nutritional standpoint, the major culprit that probably affects all these factors is a low-fiber diet.

A low-fiber diet usually results in less motility and is more likely to be associated with constipation that causes a person to strain during bowel movements. Straining causes the pressure inside the colon to increase, which is one of the major factors in diverticulum development. In contrast, a high-fiber diet produces softer and larger stool, which stimulates peristalsis and promotes regular bowel habits. In addition, in a high-fiber diet, the fiber attracts water and increases the bulk of the stool, resulting in a decrease of pressure.

A quick review of a physics principle, Laplace's law, may help. This law gives the formula for the pressure inside a cylinder, which is exactly what the GI tract represents. It states that the cylinder's pressure is equal to the tension of the walls divided by the radius (which is half the diameter) of the cylinder. So, as the radius increases, the pressure decreases, and that is what fiber does: by increasing the size of the stool, it increases the radius. Fiber may also be helpful in maintaining good colonic musculature by stimulating peristalsis.

Symptoms and Diagnosis

As mentioned, most people who have diverticulosis have no symptoms or have mild symptoms of cramping, bloating, diarrhea, or other problems with bowel movements. The opening of a diverticulum may bleed into the colon and appear in the stool; this condition is more common for diverticula in the ascending colon than in the descending colon. The bleeding occurs when feces get trapped inside the pouch and cause an adjacent blood vessel to rupture, probably sending the person to a physician to determine the cause of the bleeding. The physician would be able to see the diverticula after doing a colonoscopy (see Figure 6.2). Diverticulosis is also visible with a barium enema, or lower GI series, in which barium is instilled into the colon through the rectum and then a series of X rays is taken. Lower GI barium tests are similar in nature to upper GI barium tests, but they are not as accurate as the colonoscopy. A recent panel of experts in Europe, however, was not able to agree on which test is better for first diagnosing diverticular disease.[1]

Research Update on Diverticular Disease

One study examined the effects of dietary fiber and fiber types in relation to the risk of symptomatic diverticular disease. The subjects were a group of 43,881 American male health professionals who were free of diagnosed diverticular disease, colon or rectal polyps, ulcerative colitis, and cancer.[2] The study began in 1986, when participants completed a detailed food frequency questionnaire and information about their medical history, age, weight, height, smoking habits, alcohol consumption, and physical activity. Every two years (in 1988, 1990, and 1992), follow-up questionnaires were sent to participants so that they could update information on potential risk factors and identify newly

Q What is a colonoscopy?

A A colonoscopy is a test that uses an endoscope called a *colonoscope*, a flexible tube from 1 to five feet long and ¼ to ½ inch in diameter, to detect problems in the colon. Fiber-optic video systems provide a light source and a method for viewing; metal wires may be attached to hold clippers and an electric probe to destroy abnormal tissue. This test allows the physician to see the entire colon and even the terminal ileum, the last segment of the small intestine.

Q How is it done?

A First, the patient fasts the night before the procedure. Before the procedure, the patient uses either an enema or an oral (Colyte) preparation to clear the colon by producing diarrhea. Before the colonoscopy, the patient is sedated to minimize discomfort. During the procedure, which takes up to one hour, the patient lies in a fetal position, and a colonoscope is placed into the rectum. The colonoscope can be pushed through the entire colon and into the terminal ileum.

Q What diseases can it detect?

A A colonoscopy can detect tumors (cancerous or benign polyps), obstructions, diverticulosis, inflammatory bowel disease, hemorrhoids, and other abnormal conditions of the lower GI tract.

Figure 6.2 Common Questions about Colonoscopy

diagnosed cases of various diseases. In this study, symptomatic diverticular disease was documented in 362 cases. The findings provided evidence for the hypothesis that a diet high in dietary fiber decreases the risk of diverticular disease. This conclusion has now been verified using a variety of different techniques. The association was more significant for the insoluble component of fiber, and this inverse relationship was particularly strong for cellulose.

Insoluble fiber is the major dietary fiber fraction; it can be found in fruits, vegetables, wheat bran, whole-wheat breads and cereals, seeds, and legumes. Overall, fruits and vegetables tend to be higher in cellulose than cereals. Cellulose comprises approximately one-third or less of the total fiber in most foods, with the exception of legumes, in which it is about half.

Although dietary fibers have been divided into soluble and insoluble fractions, most foods contain both components in varying ratios.[3] Both types of fiber have been proven to be very beneficial for a variety of diseases. Insoluble fibers are considered to be those with the greatest effect on fecal bulk, which is why they are desirable for diverticular disease.

Treatment and Nutritional Intervention

When diverticulitis first develops, the symptoms are usually severe enough to send the person to the emergency room. Symptoms include moderate to severe pain and tenderness in the lower abdomen, nausea, vomiting, and fever. Rectal bleeding, from a ruptured vessel in the colon, is also possible. If a person has had diverticulitis in the past, future flare-ups, if not too severe, can often be treated at home through rest, fasting at first followed by a clear liquid diet, and antibiotics. As the symptoms subside, usually within a few days, patients follow a soft, low-fiber diet (see Figure 6.3). After four to six weeks, a high-fiber diet is recommended (see Figure 6.4). In addition, a low-fat diet may be helpful in reducing pressure inside the colon (see Figure 6.5 on pages 120–121).

In the hospital, severe diverticulitis warrants complete bowel rest, which means no food or beverages and only small sips of water or ice chips. As the inflammation subsides, the diet progresses to clear liquids. It may be necessary to provide nutritional support, either parenteral or a basic enteral formula, if the person is acutely ill and is nutritionally compromised. For most patients, antibiotics and bowel rest alleviate symptoms within two to five days. After a clear liquid, patients progress to a bland or a soft diet, with no nuts, seeds, or any fibrous vegetables.

Diet During Acute Flare-Ups of Diverticulitis Requiring Hospitalization
1. Follow a low-residue diet, or an oral elemental diet (Alitraq, Subdue); total parenteral nutrition may be required.
2. Proceed to a clear liquid diet.
3. As food is tolerated, begin a bland diet.

Diet in Cases of Acute Diverticulitis at Home
Avoid nuts, seeds, fruit and vegetable skins, fibrous vegetables, excessive fiber, highly spiced foods.

Diet for Diverticulosis (After Diverticulitis Has Subsided)
1. Consume six to eleven servings of whole-grain bread, cereals, flours, and other whole-grain products daily.
2. Consume five to eight servings of fruits and vegetables daily, especially legumes, raw fruits with skins, dried fruits, raw vegetables (carrots, celery), and vegetables with skins (potato).
3. Consume 25 grams of fiber daily.
4. Consume 2 quarts of water daily (eight, 8-ounce glasses).
5. Reduce fat intake (see Figure 6.5).

Other
1. Chew slowly and thoroughly.
2. Avoid constipation and straining.
3. Bran may be used to increase fiber intake. Begin with 1 teaspoon per day and gradually increase to 2 tablespoons daily over a one-month period to prevent cramping, diarrhea, and flatulence.
4. If fiber supplements are used, small, frequent doses are recommended. Take between meals with extra fluid two to three times per day.

Fiber Content of Foods
Beans (½ cup): 6 grams fiber
Breads, whole wheat (1 slice): 2 grams fiber
Cereals, whole grain (1 cup): 3 grams fiber
Fat: 0 fiber
Fruits, raw (1 medium): 2 grams fiber
Meat (4 ounces): 0 fiber
Milk (1 cup): 0 fiber
Vegetables, raw (½ to 1 cup): 2 to 3 grams fiber

Possible Modified Diet-Induced Deficiencies
Iron (anemia)
Protein

Figure 6.3 Dietary and Behavioral Recommendations for Diverticulitis and Diverticulosis

Breakfast

   2   packets instant oatmeal

   1   tablespoon raisins

   ½   ounce toasted wheat bran

   8   ounces skimmed milk

   1   cup fresh pineapple

Snack

   4–5 carrot sticks

   4–5 celery sticks

   2   ounces vegetable dip

Lunch

   1   4-ounce veggie burger
      whole-wheat bun

   1   slice American cheese

   ½   cup three bean salad

   1   medium plum

   8   ounces skimmed milk

Dinner

   2   corn tortillas

   ½   cup fat-free Mexican-style refried beans

   3½ ounces seasoned ground sirloin

   1   ounce cheddar cheese

   ½   cup Spanish rice
      iced tea

Snack

   1   slice sponge cake

   ¾   cup frozen berries

Calories 2,087; protein 111 g (21%); fat 55 g (24%); carbohydrate 299 g (55%); cholesterol 161 mg; calcium 1,590 mg; sodium 4,192 mg; fiber, 35 g (55%).

Figure 6.4 Sample Menu for Diverticulosis

In some cases, the patient does not show improvement, and surgery is necessary to determine if a complication has arisen. About 20 percent of patients hospitalized with diverticulitis need surgery, and 70 percent of those people do not have complications after surgery. In the other 30 percent, however, serious postsurgery complications can include bleeding, an obstruction, or fistula. Fistula, a serious complication in several lower GI diseases, represents an abnormal communication between two organs. For example, a fistula can form between the colon and the bladder, leading to intestinal contents entering the bladder and bringing bacteria, which leads to infection. This complication is more common in men than in women, and it carries a high risk for more problems or even death. Surgeries for diverticulitis complications usually involve removing the problem section of colon and reconnecting the two segments.

While in the hospital and up to a month or so after discharge, the diet is low fiber. A person recovered from diverticulitis needs to resume or begin a high-fiber diet after that month, however. Some researchers have proposed that a high-fiber diet may help prevent flare-ups and complications.[4] Patients are usually advised to avoid tiny seeds, such as poppy seeds or seeds on strawberries. Theoretically, the tiny seeds could get trapped within a diverticulum triggering inflammation. If constipation or straining to have a bowel movement is a problem, stool softeners or bulk-forming laxatives may be helpful, in addition to the high-fiber diet and adequate fluid.

IRRITABLE BOWEL SYNDROME

Irritable bowel syndrome (IBS), also called spastic colitis, is one of the most common disorders of the colon; it accounts for up to 40 percent of visits to a gastroenterologist.[5] Experts estimate that it affects 20 percent of women and up to 15 percent of men. IBS is not a disease; it

Milk and Dairy

Use

Nonfat milk or buttermilk, cheese and yogurt made from nonfat milk, fat-free cottage cheese and fat-free sour cream, fat-free coffee creamers

Avoid

Milks: whole, chocolate, 2 percent, condensed, evaporated, malted; eggnog; milkshakes; whole milk cheeses; whole and 2 percent yogurt and ice cream; sour cream; half-and-half; whipping cream

Meat, Fish, Poultry, and Eggs

Use

Up to 6 ounces of lean meat or poultry without skin daily (trim all visible fat and choose preparation methods such as baking, broiling, stewing, or simmering without adding fat); low-fat luncheon meats; meat and fish packed in water; one egg yolk daily (use egg whites or egg substitutes); low-fat cottage cheese; low-fat cheeses; dried beans or peas

Avoid

Fried or fatty meats (sausage, luncheon meats, spareribs, hot dogs, stewing hens, salt pork, poultry skins, ham hocks, pig's feet, and beef unless lean); meat and fish packed in oil; heavily marbled meats, duck and goose; more than one egg yolk per day; eggs prepared in fat; nuts or peanut butter in excess of that allowed under *Fats and Oils*

Breads and Starches

Use

Plain white or whole-grain breads, English muffins, plain rolls or buns, plain bagels and pita bread, nonfat cereals, noodles, macaroni, pasta, rice, saltines, graham crackers, matzo, melba toast, low-fat crackers

Avoid

Waffles, pancakes, muffins, biscuits, doughnuts, sweet rolls, cornbread, buttered popcorn, bread stuffing, granola-type cereals, any pasta or rice with added fat, chow mein noodles

Fruits

Use

All fruits prepared without fat, fruit juices

Figure 6.5 Low-Fat Diet

Avoid

Olives, avocados, any prepared fruit products with added fat

Vegetables

Use

All vegetables prepared without fat, vegetable juices

Avoid

Fried vegetables and vegetables in cheese or cream sauce, potato chips, fried potatoes and mashed potatoes with fat in excess of that allowed under *Fats and Oils*

Fats and Oils

Use

A maximum of three servings per day (one serving equals 1 teaspoon butter or margarine or 1 tablespoon diet margarine; 1 teaspoon oil; shortening; or mayonnaise; 2 teaspoons peanut butter; 1 tablespoon salad dressing; 1 strip crisp bacon; 8 large olives; ⅛ small avocado; 10 small nuts; ¼ cup gravy; 2 tablespoons half-and-half

Desserts and Sweets

Use

Sherbet made with skimmed milk, fruit ices, flavored gelatin, angel food cake, animal crackers, vanilla wafers, fat-free fig bars, arrowroot cookies, pudding made with skimmed milk, meringues, fat-free cookies or snacks, jelly, jam, honey, gumdrops, jelly beans, hard candy, marshmallows

Avoid

Pastries; cakes; pies; sweet rolls; desserts made with whole milk, butter, chocolate, cream, eggs, nuts, shortening, or coconut; ice cream; buttered syrups; candies with butter, chocolate, coconut, cream, nuts, or shortening; caramels

Miscellaneous and Beverages

Use

Clear soups, coffee, tea, herbal tea, soft drinks

Avoid

Cream soup, sauces, gravies, coffee or tea prepared with other than skimmed milk

Figure 6.5 *Continued*

is a collection of symptoms. Thus, some researchers describe the disease as a "junk diagnosis," one to use when no other can be made. For people with the symptoms, however, the continual GI problems may seem more than a catch-all phrase. The symptoms can vary from one person to another, but they usually include abdominal cramping and pain, bloating, flatulence, alternating bouts of both constipation and diarrhea, or any one of these symptoms.

The cause of IBS is not known, but one theory suggests that people with IBS respond in an exaggerated way to certain stimuli that would only cause a mild response if any in a person without the disorder. Possible stimuli include dietary overindulgences, emotional stress or trauma, medications, hormones, and intolerance to specific substances in foods. The physical effect that produces the symptoms is a series of abnormal contractions in the colon, almost a kinking, that alters motility and results in cramping and faulty bowel patterns. Flare-ups tend to occur when a person is awake; only rarely do they cause a person to wake from sleep.

People often confuse IBS with inflammatory bowel disease (IBD), but the similarity ends with the names, acronyms, and the organs involved. In sharp contrast to IBD, which can be life threatening, IBS is not associated with any serious complications. In addition, IBS does not interfere with nutrient absorption, unless diarrhea is fairly chronic.

Research Update on IBS

In June 1997, a two-day consensus conference was held in Kingston, Ontario, to help family physicians manage patients with IBS.[6] Fifteen family physicians, fifteen specialists, and a dietitian participated. Five internationally recognized experts in IBS presented position papers on selected topics. Their goal was to produce recommendations that were practical, user friendly, and based on the best available evidence. Some of their dietary findings are as follows.

Diet has no causal role in the development of IBS, but certain dietary items may exacerbate the syndrome, they found. Many patients with IBS believe that their symptoms are caused by food, and so they exclude many foods with little evidence of improvement. Unfortunately, there is limited scientifically valid information on the relation of diet to IBS symptoms. What is known is that meal-related symptoms are aggravating but do not correlate with any intestinal damage.

Principles of dietary management include getting foods from all the food groups. In the United States, the daily food guide pyramid is used; in Canada it is the Canada food guide. Sorbitol, caffeine, alcohol, and fat may aggravate symptoms in some individuals; if so, they should be eliminated from the diet. Lactose should only be restricted for those with proven lactase deficiency. Gradual fiber supplementation, with wheat bran or psyllium, should benefit many patients with constipation. Although stronger laxatives such as stool softeners or osmotic agents may be required in certain patients, their routine use is not recommended because they can have adverse effects and can precipitate diarrhea. With an increase in fiber, people with IBS will also need to increase their fluid intake. Fiber added in small amounts may also help reduce IBS-induced diarrhea by absorbing water and solidifying stool.[7] Products such as kaolin, psyllium, and other insoluble fiber may be used to alleviate diarrhea.[8]

The study also found that some patients become bloated or have an increase in other IBS symptoms while taking fiber. Fiber doses must therefore be adjusted to individual patient needs. On rare occasions, it may be helpful to try an exclusion diet for a very resistant case of diarrhea-predominant IBS. Referral to a dietitian is also recommended and has proven to be beneficial for many patients. Other issues addressed at the conference that need to be considered in the care of IBS are patient education, psychosocial management, and drug therapy.

It has been difficult to offer treatment or recommendations for people suffering from IBS because the cause of the disorder is unknown.[9]

Current treatment options include high-fiber diets, bulking agents, muscle relaxants, psychotherapy, and even antidepressants. None of these treatments has proven fully satisfactory. Peppermint oil has now been added to several over-the-counter remedies for symptoms of IBS. Studies show that it relaxes smooth muscle and relieves pain caused by cramps in some patients.[10] Evidence to support its use is sparse, however.[11]

To help determine the usefulness of peppermint oil, researchers reviewed all the current evidence from randomized controlled trials. Five double-blind placebo-controlled randomized trials were entered in a metanalysis, a pooling of many studies on the same topic. Overall, the researchers found a significant beneficial effect of peppermint oil compared with a placebo in the symptomatic treatment of IBS. Some studies had design flaws, however, so the reviewers did not believe that they could make definitive recommendations from the data. The authors of this review concluded that the role of peppermint oil in the symptomatic treatment of IBS is far from established. Studies have found a beneficial effect, yet that cannot be proven beyond reasonable doubt. More well-designed studies are needed to clarify the role of peppermint oil in IBS.

Both irritable bowel syndrome and lactose intolerance are common causes of gastrointestinal problems.[12] Their symptoms closely resemble each other, and the diagnoses of these diseases can be easily confused. Many controlled clinical studies have shown that symptoms attributed to lactose intolerance often occur independently of a lactose digestion problem and that subjects experience as many symptoms after ingestion of lactose-free milk as after lactose ingestion. Some authors speculate that IBS might explain some of the symptoms attributed to lactose intolerance.

In one study, 427 heathy subjects were tested for lactose maldigestion and IBS. For each subject, a lactose tolerance test was given and a bowel disease questionnaire, which diagnosed IBS according to the

Rome criteria (a standardized guideline for IBS diagnosis), was filled out. The use of dairy products and symptoms experienced after their consumption were recorded. Lactose maldigestion was found to be the primary factor explaining subjective lactose intolerance, but IBS increased the risk almost fivefold. Female subjects and the experience of symptoms other than gastrointestinal ones also increased the chance for complaints of lactose intolerance.

Studies have shown that patients with IBS report an increase in lactose intolerance, despite no increase in the prevalence of lactose maldigestion.[13] When considering possible explanations for the symptoms of lactose digesters reporting lactose intolerance, functional bowel disorders, particularly IBS, may be important. The opposite effect has also been found; many LI patients are being misdiagnosed with IBS.[14]

These studies have shown there may be problems in the diagnosis and treatment of LI and IBS. It has been suggested that the symptoms of IBS may be wrongly attributed to LI and vice versa. To help avoid unpleasant symptoms or unnecessary food restrictions, it is imperative that a proper diagnosis be made.

In recent years, hypnotherapy has been shown to be successful in the treatment of IBS. One study used six matched pairs of IBS patients and randomly assigned them to either a gut-directed hypnotherapy or a symptom monitoring control condition.[15] Those assigned to the control condition were later crossed over to the treatment condition. The results showed that hypnotherapy treatment was superior to symptom monitoring. Individual symptoms of abdominal pain, constipation, and flatulence improved significantly, and there was a considerable decrease in anxiety scores. A two-month follow-up indicated good maintenance of treatment gains.

Researchers from St. Mark's Hospital in London tried audiotaped hypnotherapy or in-person sessions on fifty-two IBS patients who had not been helped by dietary or drug therapies.[16] The researchers had already shown that in-person hypnotherapy helped improve symptoms. The results showed that the tapes worked nearly as well as individual hypnotherapy. After three months, symptoms improved in 67 percent of in-person hypnotherapy patients and 57 percent of those hypnotized by tape.

Another group of researchers from Amsterdam has treated twenty-seven patients so far with individualized hypnotherapy.[17] Of those patients, two stopped prematurely and one remained symptomatic. All other patients experienced noticeable improvement. Pain and flatulence was reduced or completely disappeared, and bowel habits normalized.

Based on data from the literature and the above studies, it appears that hypnotherapy is a valuable addition to the conventional treatment of IBS. Further research is necessary to improve knowledge on how it works and who may be sensitive to treatment.

Diagnosis and Treatment

Because IBS does not have discernible physical signs, physicians diagnose it by ruling out other lower GI diseases and on the basis of ongoing symptoms for a period of three months. Treatment centers around diet and lifestyle. Lifestyle changes emphasize establishing regular eating patterns, establishing regular bowel habits, and reducing and managing stress (see Figure 6.6). To determine if specific foods are provoking flare-ups, an elimination and reintroduction approach can be helpful. This approach typically begins by following a spartan diet of just a few bland items, then adding a few new items each day to see if the person is intolerant of any specific food. Some common problem foods or substances in food are milk and dairy products, with up to 40 percent of IBS sufferers being lactose-intolerant,[18] caffeine, alcohol, gas-forming vegetables, and wheat or yeast for some people.

1. In cases of acute irritable colon, an elemental diet may be necessary (Criticare, Subdue, Alitraq).
2. Progress to a soft, bland diet when tolerated.
3. Progress to a high-fiber diet slowly to avoid discomforts such as bloating and flatulence.
4. Avoid alcohol, black pepper, caffeine, chili powder, cocoa and chocolate, coffee, colas, garlic, red pepper, spicy foods, sugars (especially fructose and lactose), and Sorbitol.
5. Avoid gas-producing foods (apples, artichokes, asparagus, avocados, barley, beer, bran, broccoli, brussels sprouts, cabbage, carbonated beverages, cauliflower, celery, coconut, cream sauces, cucumbers, eggplant, eggs, figs, fish, fried foods, garlic, gravy, high-fat meats, honey, kohlrabi, leeks, lentils, legumes, mannitol, melons, milk, molasses, nuts, onions, pastries, peppers, pimentos, prunes, radishes, raisins, rutabaga, sauerkraut, scallions, shallots, Sorbitol, soybeans, and turnips.
6. Avoid lactose if not tolerated (see Table 5.3: Lactose Content of Foods).
7. Avoid wheat or yeast if not tolerated.
8. Common food allergies include chocolate, dairy products, wheat, yeast, and eggs.
9. Avoid excess fat (see Figure 6.5: Low-Fat Diet.).
10. Drink 2 to 3 quarts of water daily; consume 20 to 30 grams of fiber daily.
11. One tablespoon of a bulking agent, such as Metamucil, daily may be helpful. Bran may be irritating.
12. Supplement with B-complex vitamins, calcium, vitamin D, and riboflavin (if lactose is not tolerated).

(continued overleaf)

Figure 6.6 Dietary and Behavioral Recommendations for Irritable Bowel Syndrome

Dietary/Behavior Modifications
- Eat small, frequent meals.
- Eat at a relaxed pace and at regular times.
- Avoid constipation.
- Exercise regularly.
- Use of products such as Bean-O may be helpful.
- Biofeedback, relaxation, and stress reduction techniques may be helpful.
- Identify food sensitivities and omit offending foods.

Possible Modified Diet-Induced Deficiencies
- B vitamins
- Calcium
- Riboflavin
- Vitamin D

Figure 6.6 *Continued*

Dietary changes focus on eating small, frequent meals at regular and consistent times, gradually increasing fiber intake, ensuring adequate fluid intake, and avoiding any foods that cause problems. In addition to an elimination diet to find problem foods, a person with IBS can keep a food diary to record food and beverage intake and see if flare-ups are associated with certain foods. Some of the medications that physicians prescribe include bulk-forming laxatives such as Metamucil, antispasmodic drugs to help with abdominal pain (Donnatal), and tranquilizers such as Xanax.

CHAPTER 7

Inflammatory Bowel Disorders and Celiac Disease

■ · · · · · · ■

Inflammatory bowel disease (IBD) consists of two chronic diseases, Crohn's disease and ulcerative colitis, both of which produce inflammation of the intestine. These diseases tend to cause nutrient malabsorption leading to malnutrition and can cause life-threatening complications. Several aspects of the diseases are similar—indeed, it may be difficult to tell them apart—but each also has its own pattern of attack (see Table 7.1). One significant difference between the two diseases is that surgery, which is often a necessity, can cure ulcerative colitis by removing the entire colon. In contrast, surgery for Crohn's disease increases the risk for more surgeries, and the disease has no cure.

As with most chronic diseases, the cause of IBD is still a mystery, although studies have shown links to genetics, environmental toxins, infections, and autoimmune disorders. Both diseases are high in people of Jewish ancestry, although the rate is even higher in Crohn's disease. The current thinking is that a person has a genetic susceptibility, just as for diabetes, but that the condition only surfaces in response to some trigger. The trigger may be an infectious microorganism or a toxin present in food. Researchers continue to study various factors in the environment in the development of the disease.

Table 7.1 Differences Between Crohn's Disease and Ulcerative Colitis

	Ulcerative Colitis	*Crohn's Disease*
General Information		
Age of onset	15 to 30	15 to 30
Organ involved	Rectum, sigmoid colon Colon only	Ileum, small intestine Entire gastrointestinal tract
Tissue layers	Surface membrane	All layers
Distribution of disease	In segments	Continuous
Symptoms and Complications		
Cancer risk	Higher after 10 years	No increased risk
Rectal bleeding	Common	Occasional
Steatorrhea	No	Common
Diarrhea	Yes, frequent	Yes, frequent
Vomiting	Yes	Yes
Nutritional Problems		
Protein	Lost due to diarrhea, inflammation, inadequate intake	Lost due to diarrhea, inflammation, inadequate intake
Fat	No	Malabsorption
Vitamin B_{12}	No	Yes, if terminal ileum
Vitamin A, D, E, and K	Yes, medications interfere	Yes, medications interfere
Copper, zinc, selenium	Yes, losses from diarrhea	Yes, losses from diarrhea, also malabsorption
Iron	Yes, due to bleeding	Yes, if duodenum is affected, bleeding

CROHN'S DISEASE

Crohn's disease has several other names, such as regional enteritis, granulomatous ileitis, and ileocolitis, which describe its various aspects. For example, Crohn's disease can strike anywhere in the entire length of the GI tract, from mouth to anus, but it tends to have a preference for the terminal ileum, with 35 percent of sufferers having only the ileum affected. In 20 percent of people with Crohn's disease, the colon incurs the damage; in the remaining 45 percent, the disease affects both the ileum and the colon. In the section of the GI involved, the disease produces a sandlike effect of fleshy projections inside the intestine, hence the term *granulo* to describe their appearance. The granulomas, masses of capillaries and collagen, form during the healing process after a period of active inflammation. The disease is characterized by periods of remission and exacerbation (flare-up) over the years of a person's life.

More people of Jewish ancestry develop Crohn's disease, with a nine times higher rate worldwide, than people of other ancestry. Among European Jews, the disease rate is two to three times that of African or Asian Jews. In the United States, 4 of every 100,000 Americans have Crohn's disease, with men being slightly more prone to the disease than women. It generally strikes between the ages of fifteen and thirty, but there is another peak between the ages of fifty and sixty. As evidence for genetic influence, people who have family members with either form of IBD have a higher risk for Crohn's disease than those who do not.

Current theories about the cause of Crohn's disease surround the concept of autoimmune and immune dysfunction and sensitivity to substances in the environment. The GI tract is replete with immune cells that can respond to any offending substance (usually a protein called an antigen) by launching a full-blown counterattack that includes specific antibodies to attack a specific antigen, potent inflammatory compounds, and damaging oxygen radicals. Studies have suggested that proteins in food can trigger the immune response, making food allergies partly responsible. It appears, however, that this reason cannot entirely explain the disease.[1] In autoimmune diseases, the immune system cannot distinguish between a foreign antigen from outside the body and an antigen from one of its own cells. Thus, the immune response is the same as that for an outside invader: a full-blown attack but directed at the body itself.

In addition to food allergies, some researchers have proposed that dietary intake may influence the development of Crohn's disease. A 1996 Japanese study implicated a high intake of animal protein and polyunsaturated fatty acids and a low intake of omega-3 fatty acids.[2] More recently, studies have pointed to microorganisms as possible culprits in the disease.[3]

Crohn's disease begins with inflammation, and as the disease progresses, the granulomas form as the tissue goes through cycles of inflammation, damage, and healing. All layers of the intestinal tract are affected; the surface mucosa and the submucosa layers become damaged. The tissue damage causes bleeding, diarrhea, and malabsorption. Some of the complications that can arise relate to the fibrous tissue that forms, such as obstruction and stricture, which is a narrowing of the lumen due to active inflammation or scar tissue. When the intestinal contents cannot move through the lumen, the organ can rupture and cause an often fatal infection called peritonitis. The inflamed tissue can give rise to abscesses, pus-filled pockets of infection that can spread the infection to other parts of the body. Painful cracks, or fissures, can develop around the lining of the mucus membrane of the anus. Fistulae are another complication; Crohn's disease carries a high risk for mortality when a fistula occurs.

A fistula usually arises when an inflamed loop of intestine sticks to another organ or to the skin, causing erosion. The two surfaces adhere and form an abnormal conduit between the two organs. For example, if the fistula forms between the stomach or upper segment of small intestine and the colon, then as a person eats, food enters the colon before digestion and absorption of nutrients can occur. This situation quickly leads to malnutrition, to which other aspects of the disease already predispose the person with Crohn's disease. In addition, bacteria from the colon enter the stomach or small intestine and cause further malabsorption and serious infection.

Crohn's disease can bring about complications in other parts of the body besides the GI tract. During a flare-up, the disease may cause inflammation in the joints (arthritis), whites of the eyes (episcleritis), gall bladder and its ducts, spine, and other areas. In addition, Crohn's disease can cause a type of skin rash of nodules and sores that can become infected. These non-GI symptoms are more common in children, who may not even experience abdominal pain or diarrhea. In addition, children may experience fever and poor growth and development.

The nutritional problems in Crohn's disease are many and varied. When the disease attacks the small intestine, as it most often does in 80 percent of people, nutrients cannot be properly digested and absorbed. Remember that the small intestine is the major site of all digestion and absorption. Another nutritional concern is severe diarrhea, often steatorrhea from fat malabsorption, which makes food move too quickly through the system before adequate digestion and absorption.

Fat malabsorption occurs because the terminal ileum, most often the intestinal site affected, is where reabsorption of bile salts occurs. Bile is reabsorbed and recycled so that it can emulsify fats for digestion. If the level of bile salt is low, fat cannot be digested and instead is excreted in the stools. Along with the fat go the fat-soluble nutrients, such as vitamins A, D, E, and K. Bloody diarrhea is also common, and with blood loss the body loses protein and iron. In addition to direct nutrient malabsorption, people with Crohn's disease experience abdominal pain and other GI symptoms that decrease appetite and worsen after eating. These symptoms may cause a person to be afraid to eat, reducing nutrient and energy intake and further worsening malnutrition.

Symptoms and Diagnosis

With Crohn's disease, a person initially goes to a doctor complaining of chronic bouts of abdominal pain, cramping, and diarrhea. When these GI symptoms are accompanied by inflammation in joints, skin, and the eyes, the physician will probably suspect Crohn's disease. Because of the nutritional problems commonly associated with IBD, blood tests often show low blood iron (hemoglobin, hematocrit) and low albumin and total protein. Sometimes, the white blood cell level will be high, indicating active inflammation. As with Kathy's case in the beginning of Part III, it may not be possible to distinguish between Crohn's disease and ulcerative colitis even if IBD is the suspected culprit. More invasive tests, such as a lower GI (barium enema) and a colonoscopy, especially with tissue biopsy, greatly assist in both IBD diagnosis and differentiation between the two forms.

Research Update on Crohn's Disease

Enteral feeding is now an established primary therapy for active Crohn's disease. Three different types of enteral feedings are available; the main difference among them is their form of nitrogen. Polymeric diets (PDs) have intact proteins, peptide diets contain parts of proteins of variable length, and elemental diets (EDs) contain amino acids and are considered to be less allergenic than the other diets. EDs have been used extensively in patients with uncomplicated active Crohn's disease, with remission rates comparable to those of steroids. The effects of PDs remain controversial. The results of the first double-blind randomized trial to compare the therapeutic efficacy of a polymeric diet with an elemental diet were recently published. In this study, twenty-one patients with active Crohn's disease were randomized to receive either an ED or a PD. The two preparations were identical except for the nitrogen source. Patients were initially admitted to the hospital for three to four days for initiation of the enteral feeding. Feedings were provided through a nasogastric tube in which no other food or drink except for tap water was allowed. This routine was continued for four weeks, and patients were followed up weekly as outpatients. Enteral feeding was considered successful if clinical remission, determined by a variety of diagnostic criteria, was achieved. Clinical remission was obtained in eight patients receiving ED and six patients receiving PD, but this difference was not statistically significant, which may be due to the small size of the study. The treatment failed in three cases with the PD and two cases with the ED. Another two patients did not tolerate the PD feeding. Overall, enteral feeding was successful in fourteen of the twenty-one patients.

The authors concluded that enteral nutrition is effective in treatment of active Crohn's disease and that PDs are as effective as EDs in inducing clinical remission. These results indicate that the nitrogen source is probably not relevant to the therapeutic effectiveness of enteral nutrition when used as a primary therapy for Crohn's disease. The researchers believe that the fat content, particularly linoleic acid, may be of importance. The major disadvantages of EDs are their expense and patient reports of their unpalatability. The results of this study support the use of polymeric diets as primary therapy in Crohn's disease.[4]

One serious problem in Crohn's disease is that doing an intestinal resection, which may be a life-saving surgery, increases the risk for future surgery. Because the disease strikes the small intestine, too many surgeries usually cause short bowel syndrome, which in turn causes many adverse health and nutritional effects related to malabsorption of nutrients. Japanese researchers testing the use of elemental formulas in first-time surgery in Crohn's patients reviewed the medical records of seventy-three patients with Crohn's disease who had had resections between 1974 and 1996. Of the entire group of patients, thirty-two had not received an elemental diet, whereas forty-one had received an ED, before their first resection. They found that the median time period between the first disease flare-up and the first resection was 19.3 months for the group with no ED. For the ED group, the time between onset and first resection was 67.5 months. After the first resection, all patients received elemental diets. The researchers found that the need for a second resection was signficantly different when compared with the need for the first resection. They concluded that the use of an ED is effective in delaying the time between onset of Crohn's disease and the first resection. In addition, such a diet reduced the need for a second resection. They recommend using elemental formulas early in the treatment of Crohn's disease.[5]

Researchers in Canada conducted a double-blind, placebo-controlled, multicenter study of patients with Crohn's disease to determine if a lower dose of a treatment was effective in maintaining remission after the drug helps to bring about remission from a flare-up. All the patients in the study had remission after receiving a high dose of methotrexate (25 mg), an anticancer drug, given intramuscularly once weekly. For the study, patients were randomly assigned to receive either the treatment, 15 mg of methotrexate once weekly, or a placebo for forty weeks. To determine the drug regimen's effectiveness in maintaining remission, the researchers analyzed the proportion of patients who were still in remission at the fortieth week of the study. The period of remission was defined using a scoring system (150 or less) of assessment called the Crohn's Disease Activity Index. The researchers found that after forty weeks, 65 percent of the treatment group was still in remission compared with 39 percent in the placebo group. In addition, when the patients in the treatment group did suffer a relapse, only 28 percent required corticosteroid treatment (used when flare-up is signficant) compared with 58 percent in the placebo group. In addition, none of the patients in the methotrexate treatment group had a severe flare-up. Although the drug can cause significant side effects, such as nausea, vomiting, diarrhea, and hair loss, only one patient dropped out because of nausea. The authors concluded that the lower dose of methotrexate therapy (15 mg) was effective in maintaining remission in patients with Crohn's disease who enter remission after treatment with methotrexate.[6]

In yet another study, researchers tested the use of growth hormone and a high-protein diet in thirty-seven patients with Crohn's disease. They randomly assigned patients to a treatment group of subcutaneous injections of growth hormone (5 mg dose to start, then 1.5 mg per day) or a placebo group. Patients were told to increase the daily amount of protein in their diets by two and a half times the normal recommendation. Throughout the four-month study, patients continued to see their regular doctors and receive their usual treatments. To evaluate the treatment effect, researchers used the Crohn's Disease Activity Index. The results showed that scores for the index dropped significantly in the treatment group (fewer symptoms, signs of disease) compared with the placebo group. Side effects of the growth hormone treatment included edema and headache in about half the patients, but these effects usually resolved within the first month of treatment. Although the study size was small, the authors concluded that growth hormone may be a beneficial treatment for patients with Crohn's disease.[7]

Although the cause of Crohn's disease is still unknown, studies indicate that oxidative stress may be important in its pathogenesis. Several studies have reported reduced antioxidant concentrations in patient groups with active and inactive Crohn's disease compared with controls. A diminished antioxidant defense and alterations in the fatty acid profile may play a role in the pathophysiology of inflammation in this disease.

In one study, antioxidant status, disease activity, dietary intake, and fatty acid profile were assessed in twelve patients with active Crohn's disease, fifty with inactive Crohn's disease, and seventy controls. A significantly diminished antioxidant status was observed in patients with active Crohn's disease compared with patients who were in clinical remission and controls. The antioxidant defense was also depleted in patients with inactive Crohn's disease compared with controls. The dietary intake of antioxidants did not differ significantly between the active and inactive Crohn's disease patients, but that may have been due to the small study population. Analysis of the results showed that several antioxidants and disease activity were significantly associated with the plasma phospholipid fatty acid profile in Crohn's disease patients. The presence of antioxidants might influence fatty acid composition because they prevent lipid peroxidation in cell membranes. Impaired absorption of nutrients as well as increased utilization of antioxidants due to heightened oxidative stress may be contributing factors to the lower antioxidant status. Antioxidants may inhibit in vitro production of inflammatory cytokines in IBD patients. A recent study found that antioxidant status was significantly improved in patients receiving antioxidant supplementation in addition to their regular diet for three months. The finding of diminished antioxidant defense in patients with active and inactive Crohn's disease indicates that antioxidants could potentially be used in the therapy of inflammation in Crohn's disease.[8]

Polyunsaturated fatty acids (also called n-6 fatty acids) are found in animal fat. They generate compounds in the body that promote inflammation. Fish oils contain n-3 fatty acids and tend to counter inflammation. Some researchers had speculated that blood and tissue levels of different fatty acids may be relevant to flare-ups of both forms of IBD, Crohn's disease and ulcerative colitis. In one study, researchers showed a 53 percent reduction of disease activity in ulcerative colitis patients treated with n-3 fatty acids compared with only 4 percent in the placebo group.[9]

A recent study from the Netherlands compared the fat intake and fatty acid composition of blood and fat tissue in patients with Crohn's disease and a group of controls. Twenty patients with recently diagnosed Crohn's disease and thirty-two patients with long-standing Crohn's disease in remission were matched with two healthy control groups. Dietary fat was measured using a food frequency questionnaire and by obtaining an extensive diet history. The results showed no significant difference between fat intake in the Crohn's disease patients and their controls. Patients with long-standing Crohn's disease had a significantly lower percentage of n-3 fatty acids, but levels of the n-3 fatty acid precursors, linoleic and alpha-linolenic acid, were not different. This finding suggests that the abnormal n-3 fatty acid profile in Crohn's disease patients is probably the result of the disease rather than of malabsorption of essential fatty acids. Because recently diagnosed Crohn's disease patients had no differences in their fatty acid profiles, the authors suggested that disease duration may play a role in altering levels of n-3 fatty acids. This result, however, could also be the result of steroid use, commonly prescribed for IBD.[10]

Treatment and Nutritional Intervention

Treatments for Crohn's disease depend on the phase of the disease and, during a flare-up, on its severity. Most of the treatment during a flare-up revolves around countering the inflammation, treating symptoms of pain and diarrhea, and preventing stimulation and irritation of the GI tract (see Table 7.2). In addition, if infection is present, antibiotics are important aspects of therapy.

The most powerful anti-inflammatory agents are the corticosteroids. These drugs are standard treatment given intravenously if a flare-up is severe enough to require hospitalization and are taken orally for moderately severe flare-ups treated at home. Corticosteroids provide dramatic relief and induce remission, especially at high doses. Although these drugs are potent, fast-acting, and absolutely necessary for severe flare-ups, their chronic use can lead to severe side effects,

Table 7.2 Medications in the Treatment of Crohn's Disease

Problem	Medication
Diarrhea, cramping	Diphenoxylate, loperamide, deodorized opium tincture, or codeine
	Psyillium laxatives help diarrhea and constipation by firming stool
Infection	Broad-spectrum antibiotics; metronidazole (antibiotic which helps relieve Crohn's disease, especially fistulae and anal abscesses)
Inflammation	Prednisone (corticosteroids) for flare-ups; sulfasalazine, mesalamine, olsalazine (to help prevent flare-ups)

including electrolyte imbalance, weight gain, muscle wasting, bone mineral depletion, cataracts, ulcers, diabetes, and congestive heart failure. When these drugs are used, a low-sodium diet can be helpful to prevent fluid retention and some of the subsequent symptoms (see Figure 7.1).

When complications arise or when areas of tissue are severely damaged, surgery is necessary. Surgery involves removal of the affected segments of intestine and reconnecting the other two segments in a process called bowel resection. The problem in Crohn's disease is that once this life-saving surgery is performed, the need for further surgeries is increased because the disease attacks other segments. Because the small intestine is most often affected, serious health risks arise depending on how much of the small intestine was removed. The surgery causes a condition known as short bowel syndrome (see chapter 8), which is accompanied by many nutritional problems. Much of the health and nutrition risk depends on the person's health, nutritional status, and other factors, but with removal of 75 percent of the small

Milk and Dairy
Use

Milk, including yogurt (up to 16 ounces per day), buttermilk (limit to 1 cup per week), low-sodium cheeses (less than 140 mg per serving), low-sodium cottage cheese

Avoid

Chocolate milk, malted milk, milkshakes, and sweetened condensed milk; regular cheeses, cheese spreads, and cheese sauces

Meat, Fish, Poultry, and Eggs
Use

Six ounces (cooked) per day of any fresh or frozen fish, meat or poultry prepared without salt; canned fish or meats (rinsed); egg and egg substitutes (limit to one egg per day); low-sodium peanut butter or unsalted nuts; dried peas and beans processed and prepared without salt

Avoid

Salted, smoked, cured, or pickled fish meats or poultry (bacon, ham, corned or chipped beef, hot dogs, luncheon meats, meats Koshered by salting, salt pork, sausage, anchovies, herring, caviar, sardines, canned meats, crab, lobster, imitation seafood, and frozen breaded meats); pickled eggs; salted nuts

Breads and Starches
Use

Up to three slices of regular bread per day (1 slice bread, ½ bagel, ½ English muffin, ½ hamburger or hot dog bun), muffins, cornbread, and waffles without added salt; dry and cooked cereals without added salt; unsalted breadsticks, tortilla chips, pretzels, potato chips, popcorn, or crackers; barley, macaroni, noodles, spaghetti, and other pasta prepared without salt

Avoid

More than 3 slices per day of sodium-containing breads, rolls, or muffins; instant hot cereals; crackers or bread products with salted tops, salted snack foods, and salted popcorn; self-rising flour, mixes containing salt or sodium, pancakes, commercial stuffing, bread crumbs, or cracker crumbs; packaged rice or pasta dishes

Figure 7.1 Low-Sodium Diet

Fruits
Use
All fruits and juices

Avoid
Maraschino cherries

Vegetables
Use
All fresh or frozen vegetables without added salt; low sodium canned vegetables; vegetable juices without salt

Avoid
Frozen vegetables in sauces; canned vegetables with salt; packaged potato dishes and mashed potatoes with salt added; sauerkraut

Fats and Oils
Use
Margarine or butter, mayonnaise (limit to 5 servings of salted margarine, butter daily); vegetable oils and shortenings; low-sodium salad dressing; sour cream, cream, or dry cream substitutes; unsalted gravy

Avoid
More than 5 teaspoons of salted butter, margarine, or mayonnaise daily; limit regular salad dressings to 1 tablespoon daily; bacon fat, bacon bits, and salt pork; snack dips made with instant soup mixes or processed cheese; tartar sauce; gravy mixes, or canned gravy

Desserts and Sweets
Use
Not more than one serving per day of sodium-containing pudding, custard, cake, cookies, pie, or ice cream; gelatin desserts, sherbet, and fruit ice; sugar, honey, molasses, syrup, jam, jelly, marmalade, candy, and marshmallows; desserts and sweets made with milk should be within milk allowance (16 ounces per day); semi-sweet and baking chocolate; cocoa

Avoid
More than one serving per day of sodium-containing dessert; instant pudding and cake mixes; sweets containing salt; Dutch-processed cocoa; artificial sweeteners containing salt

Figure 7.1 *Continued*

Miscellaneous and Beverages
Use
Eggnog (within milk allowance), fruit juices, low-sodium or salt-free vegetable juices, low-sodium carbonated beverages, regular and decaffeinated coffee or tea and herbal tea; herbs, spices, flavoring extracts, vinegar, lemon or lime juice, hot pepper sauce, low-sodium soy sauce (1 tablespoon per day), low-sodium condiments (ketchup, mustard, chili sauce [1 teaspoon], freshly ground horseradish, and salsa [¼ cup]; vinegar

Avoid
Regular vegetable or tomato juices; commercially softened water used for drinking or cooking; salt, flavored salts (garlic salt, onion salt, celery salt, and seasoned salt), sea salt, rock salt, and Kosher salt; meat tenderizers, monosodium glutamate (MSG), regular soy sauce, barbecue sauce, teriyaki sauce, steak sauce, and Worcestershire sauce; pickles, relish, prepared horseradish and olives; meat sauces and gravies; regular condiments; flavored vinegar; salt substitutes, unless approved by a physician or dietitian

Suggestions
Omit salt in cooking and baking; try salt-free commercial seasoning and spice blends

Figure 7.1 *Continued*

intestine, the survival rate is poor. Thus, surgery points out one of the most important differences between the two types of IBD. Ulcerative colitis only affects the colon, so the entire organ can be safely removed (colectomy) without major health consequences. After removal of the colon, that disease is cured.

The many possible nutrition problems require careful monitoring and a focus on prevention. Between flare-ups in remission periods, eating an optimally nutritious diet can help prevent nutrient deficiencies and the accompanying significant nutrient malabsorption when a flare-up arises. Although a person's status of virtually all essential nutrients can become depleted, specific nutrients are special problems. Protein is likely to be a significant problem because of blood loss, and damaged intestinal mucosal tissue. All body tissues, because they are made up of cells, consist of protein so that as tissues are damaged and lost, so is protein. Because of likely poor food intake, protein can become inadequate, posing a critical problem. To repair damaged tissue and replace blood and other cells, protein is the key limiting nutrient.

Other nutrients that can become deficient include vitamins A, C, D, E, K, folate, B_6, and B_{12}, and the minerals iron, zinc, copper, calcium, potassium, and magnesium. The reasons for deficiency vary from outright malabsorption to interference from common medications. For example, the frequently prescribed sulfa drugs can cause a folate-deficiency anemia. Nutritional status can easily be imperiled by Crohn's disease. Keeping track of body weight helps to spot any unintentional weight loss that signals a suboptimal energy intake or stress from disease flare-ups quickly.

In addition to watching for likely nutrient deficiencies, other diet issues include avoiding foods to which a person may be intolerant (see Figure 7.2). Some dairy products, especially milk, can pose special problems because of secondary lactose intolerance. As small intestine tissue becomes damaged, the cells do not produce an adequate amount of lactase with which to digest lactose in most dairy products or in foods that contain dairy products. Wheat and gluten, the major protein in wheat and other grains, may pose intolerance problems for some people with Crohn's disease. In summary, careful attention to nutritional status and ensuring a nutritious diet, especially a high-protein diet, during periods of remission can help prevent nutrient deficiencies after flare-ups (see Figure 7.3).

During flare-ups, it is important to avoid excessive stimulation of the GI tract. If the flare-up is severe and the person goes to the hospital, the standard first dietary treatment is bowel rest. Bowel rest sim-

In an acute flare-up or with obstruction or fistulae

A low-residue diet, elemental diet, or total parenteral nutrition may be required.

During the acute phase of Crohn's disease
(once an oral diet is tolerated)

Avoid high-fiber foods such as nuts, seeds, fruit and vegetable skins, and fibrous vegetables; foods suspected of causing intolerance; alcohol; caffeine and caffeine-containing beverages (cocoa, coffee, cola, tea); decaffeinated coffee and tea; and pepper and spicy foods

- Reduce lactose if not tolerated (see Table 5.3: Lactose Content of Foods).
- If fat malabsorbtion exists, limit high-fat foods (see Figure 6.5: Low-fat Diet).
- Avoid wheat and gluten if not tolerated (see Figure 7.9: Dietary Recommendations for Celiac Disease).
- If corticosteroids are used in treatment, avoid excessive salt (limit to 2 grams of sodium per day; see Figure 7.1: Low-Sodium Diet).

Figure 7.2 Dietary Recommendations for Crohn's Disease

ply means that food and maybe even clear liquids are withheld for at least a short time. The theory behind bowel rest is that eliminating stimulation of the GI tract results in fewer intestinal secretions and less motility, providing a chance to recover. The concept of bowel rest is still fairly well accepted, but a newer approach is to provide minimal stimulation of the GI tract.

When the cells of the GI tract do not receive nutrients and do not do their job, they atrophy, or shrivel up. For recovery, it may therefore be more important to provide a source of nutrients that require minimal work from the intestinal cells, preventing atrophy and speeding recovery. One of the first concerns when a person is hospitalized is

Try to Eat
- 6 to 11 servings of whole-grain bread, cereals, flours, and other whole-grain products daily
- 5 to 8 servings of fruits and vegetables daily, especially legumes, raw fruits with skins, dried fruits, raw vegetables (carrots, celery), and vegetables with skins (potato)
- 25 grams of fiber daily
- 2 quarts of water daily (eight, 8-ounce glasses)
- 1 to 1.5 grams of protein per kilogram of body weight daily
- 30 to 40 calories per kilogram of body weight for adults
- 80 to 100 calories per kilogram of body weight for children; 60 to 80 calories per kilogram of body weight for teens
- Higher intake of omega-3 fatty acids from foods (fish, especially mackerel and tuna) or through supplements

Choose a vitamin and mineral supplement that includes
- Vitamins A, D, E, K, B_6, B_{12}, iron, zinc, copper, calcium, potassium, folate, and magnesium. Selenium supplementation may be needed with resections greater than 200 centimeters.

If corticosteroids are used in treatment
- Increase potassium intake (bananas, oranges, orange juice, potatoes, legumes, fruits, and vegetables).

If antidiarrheals are used in treatment
- Increase fluid intake to 2 quarts per day.

Suggested nutritional therapies include
- Antioxidants, fermentable fibers, medium-chain triglycerides (MCT oil), omega-3 fatty acids, short-chain fatty acids, and specific amino acids such as glutamine.

Commonly noted exacerbating factors in Crohn's disease include
- Increased sucrose (sugar) intake, lack of fruits and vegetables, low-fiber intake, altered n-6 : n-3 fatty acid ratios

Figure 7.3 Diet for Crohn's Disease in Remission

Dietary/Behavior Modifications
- Eat small, frequent meals.
- Chew food well. Avoid swallowing air.
- Note food intolerance and eliminate only those foods known to *consistently* cause distress.
- For extra calories, drink small amounts of an isotonic liquid oral supplement (Osmolite, Isocal) throughout the day.

Possible Modified Diet-Induced Deficiencies:
- B vitamins
- Calcium
- Fat-soluble vitamins (A, D, E, K)
- Fiber (in acute phase)
- Riboflavin
- Vitamin D

Figure 7.3 *Continued*

to treat or prevent dehydration, which is quite likely if the person was experiencing severe diarrhea. Thus, the person would receive an IV of fluids, electrolytes, and glucose.

The method for providing this source of nutrition can be either oral if the person is well enough to drink or via a tube. The formulas that serve as a source of these easily handled nutrients are called elemental, predigested, or partially hydrolyzed enteral formulas, depending on whether the nutrients have already been broken down or digested to a varying extent. For example, protein is present as short chains of amino acids and carbohydrate is glucose, which means less work for the gut. This nutrition source is called enteral, because it is delivered into the GI tract. It may be necessary, if the exacerbation is severe and the person is nutritionally compromised, to use parenteral nutrition for a time. A person with major complications, such as fistula and obstruction, will most likely need parenteral nutrition. Even so, it is important to begin to progress the diet as soon as possible. Depending on the time it takes to recover from the attack, the progression may be slow, from liquids to soft foods and then to a regular diet.

If the person's attack was not severe enough to be hospitalized but rather is treated at home, some of the same principles still apply. Fluid intake is key in preventing dehydration, and minimal stimulation is best. To achieve these goals, some people with Crohn's disease have reported some benefits of drinking elemental enteral formulas to obtain nutrients, energy, and fluid. The products are expensive, and taste may be a problem for some people. If the person is experiencing steator-rhea, foamy fat-containing stools, a lower intake of fat is usually helpful, and a special fatty acid product can also be useful. Medium-chain trigylcerides are a form of fat that do not require emulsification and minimal digestion to be absorbed. They can be used to help get the extra calories a person needs, without causing steatorrhea. A lower fiber intake is important to reduce GI stimulation (see Figure 7.4).

ULCERATIVE COLITIS

Ulcerative colitis has a similar pattern as Crohn's disease in the age of onset, typically between fifteen and thirty, with another peak between fifty and seventy years. As with Crohn's disease, but to a lesser extent, ulcerative colitis is also higher among people of Jewish ancestry, with a four to five times higher rate among this group than among other groups. In the United States, 5 to 7 Americans out of 100,000 develop ulcerative colitis. People who have had the disease for ten years have a significantly higher risk for developing intestinal cancer, in contrast with Crohn's disease, which poses no significant cancer risk.

Although symptoms are similar, ulcerative colitis appears somewhat different from Crohn's disease under the microscope. In Crohn's

Breakfast
- ¾ cup raisin bran
- 8 ounces skimmed milk (lactose reduced if needed)
- 1 slice cracked-wheat toast
- 1 teaspoon margarine
- 1 teaspoon jelly

Snack
- ½ cup unsweetened applesauce
- 2 rice cakes
- 2 tablespoons chunky peanut butter

Lunch
- 3 ounces sliced roast turkey breast
- 2 slices cracked-wheat bread
- 1 tablespoon light mayonnaise
  lettuce and tomato slice
- 8 ounces skimmed milk (lactose reduced if needed)
- 1 fresh pear

Dinner
- 3 ounces baked Atlantic mackerel
- ¾ cup mixed vegetables (broccoli, cauliflower, and carrots)
- 1 baked potato with skin
- 1 tablespoon sour cream
- 8 ounces skimmed milk (lactose reduced if needed)
- 1 banana

Snack
- ¼ cup tuna salad
- 8 Wheat Thins
- 1 orange

Calories 2,186; protein 117 g (21%); fat 67 g (28%); carbohydrate 297 g (51%); cholesterol 134 mg; calcium 1,176 mg; sodium 2,022 mg; fiber 26 g (55%).

Figure 7.4 Sample Menu for Crohn's Disease in Remission

disease, all layers of the intestine are inflamed, but in ulcerative colitis, only the first layer of the colon, the mucosal membrane, is affected. Ulcerative colitis most typically strikes the sigmoid segment of the colon, with extensive involvement of the rectum. It often spreads farther up throughout the colon so that the entire organ may be affected, but it never involves the small intestine. This fact makes the disease eventually curable, by removal of the colon. Because the main functions of the colon are to reabsorb water and electrolytes and to prepare waste for excretion, its removal has less impact on the person's health than removing sections of the small intestine. Of course, the psychological impact of colon removal is challenging for many patients.

Complications in ulcerative colitis are as severe as those for Crohn's disease. One of the most critical is toxic colitis, when the entire colon wall becomes damaged and produces a condition known as ileus, in which the organ loses its ability to move. *Ileus* means that intestinal contents are not pushed along by peristalsis. The abdomen becomes distended, the colon loses muscle tone, and soon it begins to dilate. The dilation can happen in hours or over a couple of days; when it is severe, it is called *toxic megacolon*. This condition quickly leads to perforation if not detected and treated. If perforation occurs, the risk for death is high.

Ulcerative colitis can also affect other parts of the body, much the same as Crohn's disease can. The most common problem is inflammation in other organs and tissues, such as joints, various parts of the eyes, skin nodules, spine, the liver, and the gallbladder. Bleeding is another common problem and can cause iron-deficiency anemia. In addition to anemia, other nutritional problems are general malnutrition, protein losses, electrolyte disturbances and dehydration, anorexia, and weight loss. In contrast to Crohn's disease, most of the nutritional problems are not directly due to malabsorption, but as with Crohn's disease, a person with ulcerative colitis is often afraid to eat, and the symptoms of pain and diarrhea promote anorexia.

Symptoms and Diagnosis

The typical symptoms for ulcerative colitis include chronic bloody diarrhea that persists through the night, fever, and abdominal pain (although some people do not experience pain). Lab tests usually show low albumin, iron-deficiency anemia, and a high level of white blood cells. The diagnosis is made on the basis of a sigmoidoscopy, which also indicates the disease's severity. A lower GI barium enema X ray can also show the signs of disease. The colonic tissue almost always appears abnormal, even during periods of remission.

Research Update on Ulcerative Colitis

Researchers recently tested the effect of special-formulated cereals in fifty patients with either Crohn's disease or ulcerative colitis. They designed the study to see if they could stimulate the body's production of a protein, antisecretory factor (AF), by feeding patients a cereal that had been hydrothermally processed (using a heat and water technique). Previous studies in animals had shown that the special cereal stimulates AF production. The treatment group consisted of sixteen women with an average age of fifty years, and ten men with an average age of forty-one. The placebo group was made up of twelve women with an average age of forty-one, and twelve men with an average age of fifty-one. For four weeks, the treatment group ate the special cereal and the placebo group had regular cereal. Before and after treatments, researchers assessed changes in bowel symptoms, blood levels of AF, and biopsies of colon tissue. They found that the treatment increased AF levels as they had expected and that the special cereal also significantly improved the patients' own ratings of their symptoms. The authors concluded that these hydrothermally processed cereals can increase AF levels and may improve symptoms of IBD.[11]

Treatment and Nutritional Intervention

Treatment for ulcerative colitis is similar to that for Crohn's disease, with the goals of countering the inflammation, alleviating symptoms, and correcting dehydration and nutrient deficiencies (see Figures 7.5 and 7.6). When the disease is in remission, a high-protein, nutrient-dense diet is the best approach to stave off nutritional problems when a flare-up does occur. If the disease affects the descending colon, enemas containing corticosteriods or mesalamine are often helpful to reduce symptoms. Recently, short-chain fatty acid enemas have offered a new treatment for ulcerative colitis (see Figure 7.7). The compounds appear to help in the disease by serving as an energy source for colon cells and by inducing enzymes, which promotes healing of the tissue.[12] If blood loss has been significant, it may be necessary to have a blood transfusion. A sample menu for ulcerative colitis is given in Figure 7.8.

Disease progress must be continually monitored because of the potential for cancer, for which ulcerative colitis increases the risk. When surgery is needed, diseased segments of the colon or the entire organ can be removed. Because the colon has no role in nutrient absorption, there is no concern for short bowel syndrome as with Crohn's disease. In the event of colectomy or removal of the rectum, however, a patient has to adjust to an ostomy, the creation of an artificial opening through which waste products can be excreted (see chapter 8).

CELIAC DISEASE

Celiac disease has several other aliases, including nontropical sprue, gluten-induced sprue, gluten-induced enteropathy, and gluten-sensitive enteropathy. It is characterized by malabsorption of nutrients, which is caused by genetic sensitivity of mucosal cells in the small intestine to various compounds in grain proteins. In wheat, the com-

1. Avoid foods known to cause diarrhea.
2. Avoid extremes in food and beverage temperatures (avoid iced beverages).
3. Avoid carbonated beverages.
4. Eat small, frequent meals; stop eating two to three hours before bed.
5. Eat slowly and chew well.
6. If corticosteroids are used in treatment: follow low-sodium diet; increase potassium intake (bananas, oranges, orange juice, potatoes, legumes, fruits, and vegetables).
7. Consume 2 quarts of water daily (eight, 8-ounce glasses).
8. Consume 1 to 1.5 grams of protein per kilogram of body weight daily.
9. Increase intake of omega-3 fatty acids from foods (fish, especially mackerel and tuna) or through supplements.
10. Choose a vitamin and mineral supplement that includes thiamin, vitamin E, iron, zinc, calcium, potassium, and folacin.

The following foods are suspected of causing intolerance; avoid if they have an adverse effect:

- Alcohol; caffeine and caffeine-containing beverages (cocoa, coffee, cola, tea); decaffeinated coffee and tea; pepper and spicy foods. Reduce lactose if not tolerated (see Table 5.3: Lactose Content of Foods). If fat malabsorption exists, limit high-fat foods (see Figure 6.5: Low Fat Diet). Avoid wheat and gluten if not tolerated.

During acute phases of ulcerative colitis, the following diets may be required:

- Total parenteral nutrition (when large portions of the colon are surgically removed).
- Oral elemental diet of products such as Subdue, Alitraq, or EleCare that include SCFAs, glutamine, vitamin E, and omega-3 fatty acids.

During the acute phase of ulcerative colitis (once an oral diet is tolerated):

- Follow a low-fiber diet and avoid high-fiber foods such as nuts, seeds, coarse grains, legumes, fruit and vegetable skins, and fibrous vegetables.

Possible modified diet-induced deficiencies (if lactose is not tolerated):

- Calcium
- Riboflavin
- Vitamin D

Figure 7.5 Dietary and Behavioral Recommendations for Ulcerative Colitis

Milk and Dairy
Use

All fresh, powdered, or canned milk; all plain cheeses, cottage cheese, sour cream

Avoid

Yogurt that contains nuts or seeds; cheese with nuts or seeds

Meat, Fish, Poultry, and Eggs
Use

Ground or well-cooked tender beef, ham, veal, lamb, pork, or poultry; tender steaks or chops; eggs, fish, oysters, shrimp, lobster, clams, liver

Avoid

Tough fibrous meats with gristle; smooth or chunky peanut butter; nuts; seeds; dried peas; beans; lentils

Breads and Starches
Use

All plain bread, rolls, bagels, English muffins, biscuits, pancakes, and waffles; soda, saltine, or graham crackers; pretzels; cooked cereals (well-cooked oatmeal); most dry cereals; macaroni, spaghetti, noodles, refined-flour pasta, refined rice

Avoid

Breads, rolls, or crackers made with whole wheat, bran, seeds, nuts, or coconut; cereals containing whole grain or bran; dry, coarse, wheat cereals, granola, or cereals labeled high-fiber; whole-grain pasta, wild or brown rice; popcorn

Fruits
Use

All fruit juices except prune; cooked or canned fruits except those listed under *Avoid* below

Avoid

Fresh apples, blackberries, blueberries, boysenberries, cranberries, currants, dates, figs, grapefruit, guavas, kumquats, loganberries, oranges, prunes, peaches, pears, pineapple, raspberries, rhubarb, strawberries, prune juice

Figure 7.6 Low-Fiber Diet (less than 10 grams per day)

Vegetables
Use
Strained or peeled tomatoes without seeds and vegetable juices; fresh tender lettuce; cooked or canned asparagus, beets, green or wax beans, eggplant (peeled), mushrooms, pimiento; cooked peppers, spinach, pureed or canned tomato paste or sauce (without seeds); pureed winter squash (without seeds)

Avoid
Fresh, canned, or cooked artichokes, baked beans, beet greens, broccoli, Brussels sprouts, cabbage, sauerkraut, carrots, cauliflower, collard and mustard greens; cucumbers; fresh green pepper; parsnips; peas; onion; black-eyed peas; rutabagas; pumpkin; fresh tomatoes; turnips; watercress; zucchini

Fats and Oils
Avoid
Seeds, nuts, olives, avocados

Desserts and Sweets
Avoid
Desserts or candy that contain nuts, coconut, or dried fruit; jams, preserves, marmalade

Miscellaneous and Beverages
Avoid
Beverages made from fruits and vegetables or from other foods to be avoided; soups or casseroles made with vegetables that are not allowed

Figure 7.6 *Continued*

pound is gliadin, one of two protein components of the main protein gluten which gives flour its elastic qualities. Similar compounds that cause the same reaction in other grains include hordein in barley, secalin in rye, and avidin in oats.[13] These compounds act as toxins when they come into contact with the intestinal mucosa, damaging the villi and affecting their ability to secrete digestive enzymes and

Q *What are short-chain fatty acids?*

A Short-chain fatty acids are compounds that consist of six or fewer carbons. Eating soluble fiber helps generate carbons in the colon.

Q *What do they do?*

A They increase acidity of the colon, limit the colon cells' absorption of ammonia, and promote bacterial growth in the colon.

Q *Why are they helpful?*

A Short-chain fatty acids are helpful because higher acidity in the colon lowers the breakdown of bile acids (after breakdown, they are potential carcinogens); they also protect colon cells from cancerous changes. More bacteria can then convert toxic compounds to harmless forms. Small studies have shown that enemas containing butyrate, a short-chain fatty acid, may help prevent flare-ups in ulcerative colitis.

Figure 7.7 Common Questions about Short-Chain Fatty Acids

absorb nutrients. The disease usually appears in childhood, but it may also first appear in young adulthood.

The incidence in North America is about 1 in 2,000 to 3,000. Celiac disease, however, is much higher among Europeans; in Ireland, 1 in 300 are affected. In Asia and Africa, the disease is rare. Some people are at higher risk for the disease by virtue of having a relative with the disease, but other conditions that increase its risk include Down's syndrome, type 1 diabetes, and chronic arthritis in childhood.

Nutritional problems abound because of the disease's interference with nutrient digestion and absorption. The main nutrients malabsorbed are fat, fat-soluble vitamins, minerals, protein, and carbohydrate. Celiac disease causes weight loss and anemia, and the decrease in blood protein causes edema, or fluid accumulation in the extremities. All the nutrients involved in bone health—calcium, phosphorus, magnesium, and vitamin D—are malabsorbed, producing bone disease. In addition to diarrhea, which is typical of malabsorption, fat malabsorption causes steatorrhea.

Breakfast

1	cup cream of rice (no added salt)
1	teaspoon margarine
1	tablespoon nondairy creamer
1	egg plus one egg white, scrambled
6	ounces calcium-fortified grapefruit juice

Snack

1	cup low-fat vanilla yogurt with active cultures (if tolerated)
1	cup canned peaches (juice packed)

Lunch

3	ounces low-salt tuna in water
1	tablespoon low-fat mayonnaise
2	slices white bread (if wheat tolerant)
½	cup pureed winter squash
1	cup cantaloupe pieces
1	cup calcium-fortified orange juice

Snack

1	plain bagel (if wheat tolerant)
1	tablespoon jelly
1	banana

Dinner

3	ounces broiled loin pork chop
½	cup sweet potatoes in light syrup
1	teaspoon margarine
½	cup canned green beans
1	ounce pound cake
2	tablespoons nondairy whipped topping
1	cup calcium-fortified juice

Snack

1	slice white bread
2	ounces roasted, skinless chicken breast
1	tablespoon low-fat mayonnaise

Calories 2,186; protein 117 g (21%); fat 67 g (28%); carbohydrate 297 g (51%); cholesterol 134 mg; calcium 1,176 mg; sodium 2,022 mg; fiber 26 g.

Figure 7.8 Sample Menu for Ulcerative Colitis

Symptoms and Diagnosis

Gastrointestinal disturbances, including abdominal bloating, pain, and diarrhea, are usually the first sign of celiac disease for most people. In children, the symptoms may be mild at first and may not even include diarrhea, and parents may dismiss them as simple stomachaches. Some children, however, may have more severe symptoms, especially steatorrhea, and may also begin to show signs of inadequate nutrition, with slow growth and iron-deficiency anemia. Adolescent girls with celiac disease may not have menstrual cycles.

Interesting new research shows that traditional GI symptoms may be delayed for up to eight years in some adults, with the first clinical signs being iron-deficiency anemia, bone disease, and sterility in women.[14] In the past, diagnosis of celiac disease required intestinal biopsy. Now, however, physicians can do a blood test and check for antibodies to gliadin. Another test measures the absorption of xylose, a type of sugar used as an artificial sweetener in chewing gum.

The confirming diagnosis for celiac disease, however, is a biopsy specimen that shows flattened and damaged intestinal villi and especially improvement on biopsy with the elimination of gliadin/gluten from the diet. The difficult aspect of diagnosis is making sense of symptoms that are not very specific and that can vary from one person to another.

Research Update on Celiac Disease

Italian researchers recently studied a possible link between indigestion, dyspepsia, and celiac disease. The prevalence of this disease among Italians is higher than among Americans, with 1 in 200 of the population affected. The researchers conducted upper GI endoscopy on 517 patients being seen for dyspepsia. Based on the tests, six patients were subsequently diagnosed with celiac disease, representing more than twice the risk in the general population. The authors concluded that the prevalence of celiac disease in patients with dyspepsia is twice that of the general population. They recommend that patients reporting indigestion to their physicians should be screened for the disease. Because it is easily treated when diagnosed early and because lack of treatment causes intestinal damage, physicians should consider celiac disease early in their contact with these patients.[15]

People with celiac disease are advised to follow a gluten-free diet, which entails avoiding many types of grain products. Because they no longer eat many enriched wheat products, a major source of thiamin, riboflavin, niacin, iron, and folic acid is lost from their diet. Many of the gluten-free alternatives are not required by law to be enriched.

One study was conducted to determine whether gluten-free cereal products contain similar amounts of thiamin, riboflavin, and niacin as the wheat products they are intended to replace. These nutrients were assessed because they are likely to be overlooked. Information was gathered from manufacturers, distributors, and retailers of gluten-free products. Enrichment status of 368 gluten-free products was determined. The thiamin, riboflavin, and niacin contents of 64 products were reviewed and compared with the vitamin contents of similar wheat-containing foods. The results found only 35 of the 368 gluten-free products assessed for enrichment status to be enriched. The gluten-free flours, in general, were not found to be enriched, with the exception of degermed cornmeal and corn flour, which come in both enriched and nonenriched varieties. Most bread products and all the pasta varieties reviewed were not enriched. Four gluten-free cereals made by major cereal manufacturers were enriched, but the 17 made by less well known cereal manufacturers were not. Many of the gluten-free cereal products did not provide the same level of thiamin, riboflavin, or niacin as enriched wheat products. The results showed that a gluten-free diet could potentially be lacking in one or more of the nutrients analyzed, especially if the diet consists mostly of foods that are refined and unenriched. Without dietary intake assessments, however, it cannot be concluded that adherence to a gluten-free diet actually does result in a deficiency of thiamin, niacin, or riboflavin. Recommendations for people with celiac disease include consumption of gluten-free cereals in the form of whole-grain or enriched products as well as other foods rich in these nutrients, such as legumes, nuts, seeds, green vegetables, dairy products, meat, poultry, and fish.[16]

The conventional treatment for celiac disease is the gluten-free diet, which requires the complete avoidance of wheat, rye, barley, and oats. Since the gluten-free diet was first advocated in the 1960s, there has been much debate over the toxic role of oats.[17] This controversy results from the difficulty of identifying the precise amino acid sequence in gliadin that is responsible for the toxicity. A growing body of evidence now suggests, however, that moderate amounts of oats may be safely consumed by most adults with celiac disease.[18]

A recent study has found that oats do not harm intestinal villi in adults with celiac disease.[19] The researchers compared the immunological effects of a gluten-free diet including oats with a conventional gluten-free diet. Forty adults with newly diagnosed celiac disease and fifty-two with the disease in remission were examined in a randomized control intervention study over six to twelve months. The measures of immunological function were found to be the same between the two groups. The authors concluded that adult patients with celiac disease can consume moderate amounts of oats without adverse immunological effects.

One case-control study suggested that inclusion of a purified oat product in a gluten-free diet does not prevent healing of the intestine or alter outcomes compared with a diet that excludes oats.[20] In this study, however, a specially grown and tested oat product was used; the results may not be applicable to commercially obtained oats, which may be subject to contamination in the field or in processing.

What recommendations on the use of oats in a gluten-free diet are being made to persons with celiac disease? A questionnaire on the acceptability of several foods was mailed to United States and foreign celiac organizations and to physicians treating people with celiac disease. With regard to oats, only five of thirty-three respondents considered them acceptable in a gluten-free diet. Many respondents had concerns about the possible toxicity of oats, either directly or indirectly by contamination. Other reasons were insufficient research and lack of information on the amount of oats that may be safely consumed.[21]

Although some experts appear optimistic about the safety of oats, others believe that it is premature to begin recommending oats to patients with celiac disease.[22] The Gluten Intolerance Group of North America, among others, continues to recommend the complete avoidance of oat products. Advice about oats tends to vary, however. Some hospitals in Canada, for instance, have previously allowed the consumption of oats by their patients with celiac disease.

There is still a need for consensus between celiac organizations and physicians about appropriate foods for inclusion in a celiac patient's diet.[23] If further research continues to find no adverse effects from oats consumption, a consensus may emerge on including oats in the gluten-free diet.[24] Allowing oats can improve the nutritional quality of the diet and increase food variety for people with celiac disease.

Treatment and Nutritional Intervention

The treatment for celiac disease is elimination of gliadin/gluten from the diet (see Figures 7.9 and 7.10). It is important to diagnose celiac disease and eliminate the toxin as soon as possible, because continued ingestion leads to extensive damage of the intestine. Some people with either a more severe or long-standing case may not respond to dietary

Dietary Guidelines

1. Celiac disease requires total avoidance of gluten: wheat, oat, rye, and barley.
2. Allowable foods include corn flour, cornmeal, corn starch, rice, rice flour, potato flour, soybean flour, tapioca, sago, arrowroot, gluten-free wheat starch, and lima bean flour.
3. Obtain 1 to 2 grams of protein per kilogram of body weight daily (about 80 to 120 grams for adults).
4. Obtain 35 to 40 calories per kilogram of body weight daily.
5. A multivitamin and mineral supplement (iron, folate, vitamin B_{12}, calcium, vitamin A, vitamin D, vitamin K, thiamin, and B-complex vitamins) should be taken.
6. Reduce lactose intake (slowly increase lactose intake to tolerance).
7. Reduce fiber intake (slowly increase fiber intake to tolerance).

Tips

- Read labels carefully and frequently. Watch for ingredients labeled hydrolyzed vegetable protein (HVP) vegetable gum, vegetable starch, vegetable protein, flour, cereal, cereal products, malt, malt flavoring, starch, gelatinized starch, modified starch, modified food starch, fillers, natural flavoring, soy sauce, soy sauce solids, monoglycerides, and diglycerides.
- Be sure to identify specific thickening agents, emulsifiers, and stabilizers.
- When dining out, inquire about special or secret ingredients and preparation methods.

Baking Tips

The following may be substituted for 1 cup of wheat flour in baking:

- 1 cup corn flour
- 1 cup coarse cornmeal (mix with liquid in recipe and boil; cool, then add to other ingredients)
- 1 cup fine cornmeal
- ⅝ cup potato flour
- ⅞ cup rice flour (mix with liquid in recipe and boil; cool, then add to other ingredients)

Figure 7.9 Dietary Recommendations for Celiac Disease

- When using soy flour, combine with another flour for best results.
- The leavening used with nonwheat flours must be increased (i.e., use 2 teaspoons of baking powder for each cup).
- Nonwheat flours require longer, slower cooking times.
- Better texture may be obtained by baking foods such as biscuits and muffins in small sizes.
- To prevent excessive dryness, store baked goods in an air-tight container.

For thickening, the following may be substituted for 1 tablespoon flour:

- ½ tablespoon arrowroot starch
- ½ tablespoon cornstarch
- ½ tablespoon potato starch
- ½ tablespoon rice flour
- 2 teaspoons quick-cooking tapioca

Foods to Avoid in Celiac Disease

Breads, Cereals, and Grains
- Gluten; wheat; whole-wheat flour; enriched flour; soft wheat flour; high-gluten flour; high-protein flour; all flour containing wheat, oats, rye, or barley; bran; graham; wheat germ; malt; kasha; bulgar; spelt; kamut; triticale; couscous; farina; seitan; semolina; durum; durum flour; groats; millet; whole-wheat berries; wheat starch; commercially prepared mixes for biscuits, cornbread, muffins, pancakes, and waffles; pasta; regular noodles; spaghetti; macaroni; most packaged rice dishes; bread crumbs, cracker meal, pretzels; matzo; gelatinized starch (may contain wheat protein)

Milk and Dairy
- Malted milk, Ovaltine, any cheese product containing oat gum, chocolate milk with cereal additive, some sour cream, some yogurt, some nondairy creamers
- If lactose tolerance is altered, see lactose intolerance diet (Figure 5.3)

Figure 7.9 *Continued*

Meat, Fish, Poultry, and Eggs

- Meats prepared with wheat, oats, rye, or barley (bologna, chili, hot dogs, luncheon meats, and sandwich spreads); creamed meats, breaded or bread-containing products (i.e., croquettes, Swiss steak, and meat loaf); meats injected with hydrolyzed vegetable protein; tuna in vegetable broth; meat or meat alternatives containing gluten stabilizers; eggs in sauces with gluten

Fruits and Vegetables

- Breaded or creamed vegetables, or vegetables in sauce; some canned, baked beans; some commercially prepared vegetables and salads; thickened or prepared fruits; some pie fillings

Fats, Oils, and Sweets

- Some commercially prepared salad dressings; some commercial candies; chocolate-coated nuts; commercial cakes, cookies, pies, and doughnuts made with wheat, rye, oats, or barley; prepared dessert mixes including cookies and cakes; puddings thickened with wheat flour; ice cream or sherbet with gluten stabilizers; ice cream containing cookies, crumbs, or cheesecake; ice cream cones

Alcohol

- Ale, beer, gin, whiskey, vodka distilled from grain

Miscellaneous

- Herbal teas with malted barley or other grains with gliadin (see *Breads, Cereals, and Grains* list above); most canned soups, cream soups, and soup mixes, bouillon; some curry powder; dry seasoning mixes; gravy extracts; meat sauces; catsup; mustard; horseradish; soy sauce; chip dips; chewing gum; distilled white vinegar; cereal extract; cereal beverages (Postum); root beer; yeast extract; malt syrup; malt vinegar; commercial infant dinners with flour thickeners; caramel color and monosodium glutamate (may not be tolerated)

Figure 7.9 *Continued*

Breakfast

1½ cups puffed rice cereal

8 ounces 2 percent milk (lactose reduced if necessary)

1 banana

8 ounces orange juice

Snack

1 ounce dry-roasted peanuts

1 mozzarella cheese stick (1 ounce)

Lunch

3½ ounces lean ham

½ cup sliced carrots

½ cup wild rice

8 ounces 2 percent milk

½ cup fruit cocktail (in juice)

Dinner

3½ ounces broiled sirloin steak (fat trimmed)

1 baked potato

½ cup steamed broccoli

2 teaspoons soy margarine

8 ounces 2 percent milk

1 cup strawberries

Snack

2 cups microwave popcorn

Calories 1,943; protein 108 g (22%); fat 66 g (31%); carbohydrate 240 g (47%); cholesterol 198 mg; calcium 1,330 mg; sodium 3,044 mg.

Figure 7.10 Sample Menu for Celiac Disease

intervention. In this situation, corticosteroids can usually bring about improvement. For adults with an even more severe form of celiac, the disease can be fatal. One complication of celiac disease in adults is the development of lymphoma of the intestine. Lymphoma is cancer of the lymphoid tissue, which is tissue that connects a certain type of white blood cell, the lymphocytes. Experts do not yet know if a gluten-free diet reduces the cancer risk.

The most obvious sources of gluten in the diet are foods that contain wheat, oats, rye, and barley; dietitians remember this list by its acronym, WORB. Although it would seem easy to avoid these grains, it is not. Wheat is a diet staple in many parts of the world; most breads and baked goods are wheat-based, even when they contain other grains. Once wheat, oats, rye, and barley are eliminated, the choices remaining are few: rice, soy, potato, and corn. Perhaps the trickiest part of the diet, however, is checking food labels for ingredients made from parts of one of the grains. For example, pick up a package of just about anything and see if any of its ingredients is on just this short list of problem substances: cereal, starch, flour, thickening agents, emulsifiers, stabilizers, hydrolyzed vegetable proteins, caramel coloring, and monosodium glutamate (MSG).

With celiac disease, as with inflammatory bowel disease, damage of the intestinal tissue may necessitate the removal of the affected sections of the small intestine. As with Crohn's disease, nutrition becomes a concern because of the small intestine's role in nutrient digestion and absorption. In contrast to Crohn's disease, however, removal of the toxin from the diet should preclude further need for surgery. If a sufficient amount of the small intestine is removed, short bowel syndrome may result (see chapter 8).

CHAPTER 8

Intestinal Surgeries

■ · · · · · · ■

Several of the diseases from the previous chapters, and intestinal cancer, may necessitate intestinal surgery. Surgery involves removing a diseased or damaged segment in either the small intestine or the large intestine and then reconnecting the other two segments in a process called resection. Such surgery can either present many nutritional problems or virtually none, depending on three key factors. The most important factor is how much intestine is lost. Although research has enabled surgeons to make great strides in treatments and surgical approaches, including a recent intestinal transplantation, removing more than 40 percent of the small intestine produces nutrient malabsorption. Malabsorption from this cause is a condition known as short bowel syndrome, and removing more than 75 percent of the small intestine is associated with a poor survival rate.

Another important factor that influences the likelihood of nutritional problems after surgery is the location of the resection. For example, the entire large intestine can be safely removed without adversely affecting nutritional status. As mentioned in chapter 7, a colectomy presents many challenges and lifestyle adjustments but, fortunately, no health effects. The surgery, an ostomy, creates an artificial opening for excretion of waste. In the small intestine, because some nutrients are absorbed in specific segments, there may be problems for a particular nutrient if its absorptive area was removed.

The terminal ileum is the absorption site of vitamin B_{12} and bile salts. As a consequence, removal of this segment will cause B_{12} deficiency, fat malabsorption, and all the problems that go along with it. The ileocecal valve is a special flap that separates the small intestine from the colon. It controls movement of the contents of the small intestine into the colon and therefore helps control transit time. If this structure is removed, bacteria from the colon can move up into the small intestine, causing severe and life-threatening diarrhea.

The third factor that affects nutritional problems after surgery is the adaptive ability of the remaining bowel. As with the human body in general, the intestine shows a breathtaking ability to come back up after the count. After intestinal tissue is removed, the remaining tissue picks up the extra duties of digestion and absorption, but the adaptive abilities of each person's intestine are unique. Researchers have identified four important determinants of intestinal adaptability: the type and location of the resection, the patient's age, the patient's nutritional status, and the content of the diet. The first two cannot be changed, but the nutritional determinants can be improved. Researchers continue to learn more about various dietary substances that can accelerate healing and the remaining intestine's ability to adapt.

OSTOMIES

When a person has surgery to remove sections of the colon, it may be necessary to create an artificial opening for waste excretion. In a colostomy, part of the colon, the rectum, and the anus are removed, and the remaining segment of colon is brought out through the abdominal wall and forms the opening called a stoma (see Figure 8.1). An ileostomy involves a colectomy, in which the entire colon, the rectum, and the anus are removed and the ileum is brought through the opening. These procedures may be done on a temporary basis to allow healing of the colon

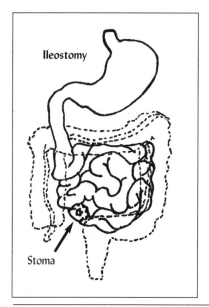
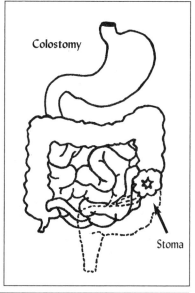

Figure 8.1 An ileostomy and a colostomy. The dotted portions indicate the removed sections.

after surgery, as in the case of colon cancer. If they are permanent, however, the person will have to wear an appliance, a plastic device with a seal between the skin and the collecting bag, to cover the stoma. Over time, the stoma shrinks to about the size of a nickel.

Adjusting to an ostomy can be a major challenge for some people. In addition to the physical adjustments relating to developing bowel regularity, the psychological impact can be difficult. It is helpful for an ostomy patient to meet with others who have had the procedure and get the support of people sharing a similar experience. Health care specialists trained in working with ostomy patients are called enterostomal therapists. Initially, specific nutritional problems and concerns may arise, depending on which procedure the patient has had. Of the two procedures, the ileostomy causes more problems because of the special absorptive role of this portion of the small intestine. In addition to nutritional problems, diet can influence various aspects of bowel regularity and stool consistency.

At one time, all patients had to wear an appliance, but more recently new procedures make it possible to avoid it. Folds of the ileum are brought together to create an ileal pouch, which the surgeon then connects to the rectum and the ileum. Interestingly, the pouch soon becomes inhabited by bacteria, just as in the colon. This step is good for intestinal health, because the bacteria provide vitamin K and keep other bad bacteria at bay. Also, bacteria are helpful because they produce short-chain fatty acids and vitamin K. On the negative side, they compete for vitamin B_{12}, so injections of that vitamin may be necessary. The pouch may also bring complications, such as obstruction, pouchitis (inflammation of the pouch), and gas. The person will have more frequent bowel movements, up to eight a day, because the pouch is smaller than the colon. Reducing caffeine intake can help cut down on possible diarrhea. To prevent obstruction, the person with an ileal pouch should chew food thoroughly, especially fibrous fruits and vegetables, and eat small, frequent meals. Pouchitis is somewhat similar to the inflammation of ulcerative colitis, probably involving only the mucosal membrane. Although researchers don't know what causes pouchitis, it's most likely the result of overgrowth of certain types of bacteria, and other possibilities include a low level of short-chain fatty acids.[1] The problem is usually treated with antibiotics, and ongoing research is looking at alternative treatments.

Ileostomy

An ileostomy produces a watery stool because with the loss of the colon, fluid is not effectively reabsorbed from the waste as it moves through the GI tract. Adjustment to ileostomy is therefore more of a

1. A clear liquid diet follows surgery.
2. Progress to a bland, low-fiber diet with extra calories (35 to 45 kcal/kg/day) and protein (1.5 g/kg/day) for healing.
3. Continue with low-fiber diet. Use sources of pectin such as oatmeal and applesauce.
4. Choose a vitamin and mineral supplement with vitamin B_{12}, folacin, calcium, magnesium, iron, and vitamin C.
5. Supplement sodium and potassium.
6. If Prednisone is used in treatment, limit salt intake (see Figure 7.1: Low-Sodium Diet).
7. Avoid eating before bedtime.
8. See additional guidelines (colostomy recommendations).

Possible Modified Diet-Induced Deficiencies
- Vitamin C
- Depends on food tolerances

Figure 8.2 Dietary Recommendations for Ileostomy

challenge than adjustment to colostomy (see Figures 8.2 and 8.3). In addition, the ileostomy will most likely cause malabsorption of fat because bile is not adequately reabsorbed. Whenever fat is not absorbed, other nutritional problems accompany the malabsorption. Vitamin B_{12} will not be absorbed because it is absorbed in the last portion of the small intestine, which is removed in the ileostomy.

Fat-soluble vitamins will also be malabsorbed, so it is important to consider a supplement, especially if a significant portion of small intestine was lost. The risk for both kidney stones and gallstones increases with steatorrhea, so it is important to monitor for and counter the development of these conditions. The most important prevention is adequate fluid intake. It is also prudent to avoid foods high in oxalate, such as spinach, rhubarb, wild greens, coffee, tea, and chocolate. An ileostomy also causes excessive fluid losses along with electrolyte loss, making dehydration a special concern.

Breakfast

2   packets instant oatmeal
1   tablespoon brown sugar
1   tablespoon nondairy creamer
6   ounces cranberry juice

Snack

½   cup unsweetened applesauce
½   cup low-fat cottage cheese

Lunch

2   slices whole-wheat bread (white bread with ileostomy)
2   ounces baked ham
1   ounce slice American cheese
1   teaspoon low-fat mayonnaise
1   banana

Snack

8   ounces low-fat lemon yogurt
½   cup canned pears (packed in juice)

Dinner

3½   ounces roasted round steak (fat trimmed)
¼   cup gravy
½   cup mashed potatoes
½   cup canned carrots
½   cup canned peaches (packed in juice)

Snack

2   tablespoons smooth peanut butter
7   Triscuits
½   cup calcium-fortified juice

Calories 2,079; protein 97 g (19%); fat 59 g (26%); carbohydrate 290 g
(55%); cholesterol 151 mg; calcium 1,115 mg; sodium 3,962 mg; fiber 26 g.

Figure 8.3 Sample Menu for Ileostomy

Gassiness can also be a problem, and avoiding cruciferous vegetables, legumes, and other potential gas-forming fruits and vegetables may be helpful. If enough gas builds up, the appliance can become dislodged. Steatorrhea and gas are also associated with odor, although deodorant pills and odor-proof pouches are now available. People with ileostomies begin to identify specific foods that cause odor problems. Most of the foods are similar to those causing gas, but others include corn, fish, highly spiced foods, and medications such as antibiotics and vitamin-mineral supplements. Another source of odor is inadequate hygiene of the stoma, and the enterostomal therapist can help in this area.

Obstruction is another possible complication, so it is important to chew food well, especially fibrous items. Over time, the small intestine adapts, and many problems and concerns improve as the organ has a chance to recover. The diet needs to change over this period of recovery and adjustment, from a more conservative diet immediately following surgery to as close to a regular diet as possible for the long term.

Colostomy

With a colostomy, the stool consistency is close to normal or is normal, depending on how much of the colon is removed. If the colostomy is on the right side, the stool will be mushy, whereas a left-sided colostomy produces a firm stool. Odor is a significant problem for the person with a colostomy, and attention to specific foods that cause odor problems is important. Because potential odor-causing foods are nutrient dense, it is better to focus on other approaches, such as deodorizers. Many of the same diet recommendations for an ileostomy apply to a colostomy, although the possible nutritional problems are more likely with an ileostomy (see Figure 8.4).

1. A clear liquid diet follows surgery.
2. Progress to a bland, low-fiber diet with extra calories (35 to 45 kcal/kg/day) and protein (1.5 g/kg/day) for healing.
3. After approximately two weeks, gradually increase fiber intake. Fiber intake may be adjusted if diarrhea results.
4. The following foods should be avoided only if they consistently cause undesirable effects:

May Cause Obstructions
Bamboo shoots, bean sprouts, celery, citrus fruit membranes, coconut, coleslaw, corn, fruits with skins and seeds, green beans, lettuce, mushrooms, nuts, peas and pea pods, popcorn, potato skins, raw carrots, raw and dried fruit, relishes, seeds, spinach, tough meats, and vegetables

May Cause Odor or Gas
Antibiotics, asparagus, beer, broccoli, Brussels sprouts, cabbage family vegetables, carbonated beverages, cauliflower, corn, cucumbers, deep-fried foods, dried beans and peas, eggs, fish, melons, milk, mustard, nuts, onions, pastries, pickles, radishes, some vitamin and mineral supplements, spicy foods, strong-flavored cheeses, turnips

May Contribute to Diarrhea
Beans, beer and wine, broccoli, coffee, fresh fruits and vegetables and their juices, green leafy vegetables (especially spinach), highly spiced foods, licorice, prune juice

5. Avoid high-oxalate foods (see Figure 8.5: Dietary Recommendations for Short Bowel Syndrome).
6. Applesauce, bananas, boiled milk, cheese, milk, peanut butter, rice, and tapioca may reduce diarrhea. Reducing fluid intake does not reduce diarrhea and may cause dehydration.
7. If Prednisone is used in treatment, reduce salt intake to 2 to 3 grams daily (see Figure 7.1: Low-Sodium Diet).
8. Consume 1 to 2 quarts of fluid daily, between meals.
9. Choose a vitamin and mineral supplement with vitamin E, folacin, calcium, magnesium, iron, vitamin C, vitamin K, and vitamin B_{12}.

Figure 8.4 Dietary Recommendations for Colostomy

Dietary and Behavior Modifications

- Establish regular meal times.

- Eat slowly and chew thoroughly with mouth closed.

- To prevent excess gas, avoid chewing gum or drinking from straws.

- Use cranberry juice, yogurt, buttermilk, and fresh parsley (as tolerated, in limited amounts) as natural deodorizers.

- Use products such as Bean-O to reduce gas.

- If a food has been eliminated from the diet due to diarrhea, constipation, odor, or gas, retest tolerance after two to three weeks.

Figure 8.4 *Continued*

SHORT BOWEL SYNDROME

When 40 percent or more of the small intestine is removed in a resection, short bowel syndrome is a prime concern, especially if the terminal ileum and ileocecal valve were removed. The nutritional problems associated with short bowel syndrome arise from malabsorption (see Table 8.1). The extent of the nutritional problems depends on the extent and location of the resection and the adaptive ability of the remaining intestine. Although the survival rate declines as more of the small intestine is removed, if the ileum and ileocecal valve remain intact, even an 80 percent resection can prove to be tolerated.[2] Because of its importance in long-term survival and because it is the only controllable variable, enhancing the small intestine's ability to adapt is the focus of much current research.

A person who has short bowel syndrome will experience diarrhea, steatorrhea, weight loss, muscle wasting, bone disease, and malabsorption of several nutrients, which can lead to nutrient deficiencies such as anemia. Nutrition is the key to recovery and to enhancing the

Table 8.1 Malabsorption in Short Bowel Syndrome

Deficit/Problem	Result
Bile acid	Fat not digested, bacterial overgrowth
Absorptive surface	Maldigestion, malabsorption
Fluid reabsorption	Dehydration
Increased motility, short gastrointestinal tract	Dumping syndrome
Loss of ileocecal valve	Bacterial overgrowth
Oversecretion of gastric acid	Damage to duodenal tissue, pancreatic enzyme activity altered
Pancreatic enzyme activity	Maldigestion, malabsorption
Fat malabsorption	Kidney stones, gallstones

small intestine's adaptive ability. One of the most crucial findings over the past several years is that early feeding, as soon as possible without damaging the small intestine, is beneficial. Historically, surgeons believed that the gut needed time to recover and that feeding anything would stimulate intestinal secretions and slow recovery. They used parenteral nutrition for extended periods. What they did not know was that minimal stimulation is actually good for the recovering gut. The trick with early feeding is knowing how early, what, and how much.

Resections of the jejunem initially cause malabsorption because most nutrients are digested and absorbed within the first 40 inches of the small intestine. After the adaptation period, however, the ileum takes over this function and can do quite well. When a significant amount of the ileum, especially the terminal ileum, is lost, though, severe nutritional and other health problems arise. Conventional wisdom and logic also suggest that the colon is expendable, and compared with the small intestine, that is certainly true. Researchers, how-ever, have shown that after resection, an intact colon may help reduce the usual malabsorption of carbohydrate and protein.[3]

During the adaptation period, the remaining intestine begins to grow in length, diameter, and thickness. A look under a microscope at intestinal villi before and after adaptation shows that the villi become longer, with deeper valleys between each, and that the number of cells on the villi increases. The result of these physical changes is an increase, to some extent, in the absorptive surface area to compensate for the intestine that was lost.

Research Update on Short Bowel Syndrome

Researchers at the University of Pittsburgh Medical Center have been busy convincing fellow researchers and gastroenterologists that intes-tinal transplants are beyond the experimental stage. Previously, the removal of most of the small intestine was a death sentence. The advent of parenteral nutrition saved many lives, but in addition to the dra-matic impact on quality of life, the feeding method can cause infection and fatal liver failure. The researchers performed their first intestinal transplant in 1990, and in 1999 they reported on the follow-up with their first patients, many of whom were young children. Of their 109 transplant patients, 72 percent were still alive one year after the surgery and 48 percent survived for five years. The transplant carries many risks, including tissue rejection, complications from powerful drugs to prevent rejection, nervous system abnormalities, lesions in blood ves-sels, and loss of blood and oxygen to the brain. Of the 175 children who did not have the transplant, the survival rate was 18 percent. Chil-dren under the age of one year had the poorest prognosis. The pres-ence of liver dysfunction was associated with poor survival. The authors concluded that intestinal transplantation should be considered a viable procedure, and that, to improve the chances of survival, it should be considered before signs of liver failure are apparent.[4]

Intestinal transplantation is moving from an experimental stage toward recognized treatment. In addition to the medical challenges, however, nutritional concerns can present problems. Currently, colon transplant is not viable, because the procedure is associated with a high risk for death because of the high level of bacteria in the colon. Patients who receive a small intestine only have the best chance for survival, especially those aged two to eighteen. The use of potent immunosuppression drugs has made transplant possible, but these drugs also cause numerous nutritional side effects. The current drug used for intestinal transplant, FK506, is an antibiotic from a fungus; it causes hyperkalemia (high potassium in blood), anorexia, and chronic high blood pressure. The drug can also damage the kidneys, pancreas, and nervous system. Another nutritional problem is when the transplant organ is stored in a cold environment. This waiting period damages the organ, and when the wait is long, the intestinal villi are destroyed, reducing the nutrient absorption ability of the organ.

After the transplant organ is placed in the recipient, the surgeon must infuse the organ with blood, causing injury to the intestinal membrane from free radicals generated from the oxygen. The procedure itself makes the organ unable to conduct normal peristalsis for up to four months. During this time, motility and transit time may cause problems. Another complication is nerve damage to the organ, which can overwhelm nutrient absorption ability. Patients often experience diarrhea for up to three months after the transplant, depleting fluid and electrolytes. If the body begins to reject the organ, the intestinal function is damaged, making fat malabsorption likely.

Many of the patients who are awaiting transplant are already nutritionally compromised from previous disease, surgery to treat the disease, or long-term parenteral nutrition. Therefore, it is important to carefully assess the patient's nutritional status and, if necessary, improve it before transplant surgery. Glutamine has been useful in promoting gut health after transplant, as have soluble and insoluble fiber. Insoluble fiber helps reduce the risk of infection and soluble fiber helps to restore function to the intestinal villi. The nutrition approach for transplant is similar to that following intestinal resections. Parenteral nutrition begins twenty-four to forty-eight hours after transplant. As soon as the gut begins to move, tube feedings begin alongside the parenteral nutrition. When 50 percent of energy needs can be achieved with tube feeding, the parenteral solution is reduced. When oral intake is possible, the diet is low fat, low lactose for four to six weeks after surgery, and tube feeding continues until oral intake is adequate.[5]

Short bowel syndrome usually results after bowel resections for Crohn's disease. Less commonly, it results from extensive small bowel diseases such as scleroderma, visceral myopathy, or neuropathy. The normal human small intestinal length ranges from about 3 to 8 meters; therefore, if the initial small intestinal length is short, a relatively small resection of the intestine may result in the problems of a short bowel. Physicians in clinical practice encounter two types of patients with short bowel syndrome: those with their jejunum connected to a functioning colon and those with a jejunostomy. Patients with short bowel syndrome have problems absorbing adequate macronutrients and need long-term vitamin B_{12} therapy.

Most patients who have less than 100 centimeters of small bowel remaining and who are maintained on oral supplements absorb only about 50 to 60 percent of their oral energy intake. They therefore need to consume twice as much energy as before the resection. Most patients can do so by eating more food, although some may use a nocturnal nasogastric tube feeding or use tube feeding during the sleep hours. Patients who have a short bowel and an intact colon should eat a diet high in carbohydrates; when carbohydrate is not absorbed by the small intestine, bacteria in the colon ferment it and produce short-chain fatty acids. The colon cells can absorb the short-chain fatty acids, providing an important source of additional energy. Fat may worsen diarrhea by reducing water and sodium absorption and increasing the transit time in the colon. Undigested fat is toxic to bacteria, so when it enters the colon it reduces the amount of carbohydrate fermented. Patients with short bowel syndrome who have an intact colon need a large total energy intake with a diet high in carbohydrates (polysaccharides) but relatively low in fat and oxalate, to help prevent kidney stones. Calcium supplements may also be helpful, as it is lost due to oxalate and fat malabsorption.

Patients with a jejunostomy absorb a constant proportion of protein, energy, and fat from their diet. Increasing fat in the diet does raise fat excretion, but the fat does not increase stool frequency and does not contribute to odor problems. These patients need a diet that is high in total energy, relatively high in fat, and with added salt due to losses.

In patients with short bowel syndrome, the rate and extent of adaptive capacity of the remaining small intestine determines the recovery period and requirement for extended parenteral nutrition.[6] Nutrients, hormones, and growth factors present in the gut can all theoretically affect intestinal adaptation. The research, however, has not been clear on the actual benefit of these compounds. Although some studies have shown conflicting results, therapy with growth factors (growth hormone, glutamine, fiber, and epidermal growth factor) have shown some success in maximizing intestinal adaptations.[7] One researcher showed benefits of combining glutamine, growth hormone, and a modified diet.[8] Studies have shown that glutamine accelerates healing after bowel resection and decreases diarrhea by enhancing sodium and water reabsorption. This therapy continues to be successful.

Treatment and Nutritional Intervention

Treatment of short bowel syndrome focuses on managing symptoms and enhancing intestinal adaptation. Several medications are useful in managing the symptoms of diarrhea, steatorrhea, and bacterial overgrowth. Drugs that slow gastric emptying and intestinal motility can help control diarrhea and thereby increase nutrient digestion and absorption. The goals of nutrition therapy are similar to the overall plan, but an additional key point is to improve nutritional status, which goes a long way in preventing nutritional symptoms and enhancing intestinal adaptation.

If 50 percent or less of the small intestine was removed, feeding can begin within a few days after surgery (see Figure 8.5). For higher resections, parenteral nutrition is the first method of feeding. If the patient has become nutritionally compromised because of the disease state that necessitated the surgery, this parenteral nutrition support is vital, and it must provide enough energy and nutrients to allow the regain of weight and nutrient stores. As soon as possible, however, enteral feedings should start because they begin to stimulate adaptation. Depending on the extent of the resection, parenteral nutrition may need to continue from three weeks to six months. The timing of the different dietary changes is variable, and it may be months before a person can eat normally again. In the meantime and along with parenteral nutrition, enteral feeding can begin with a small volume, gradually increasing in volume over the next weeks. The enteral feeding should be an elemental formula, partially predigested, so that the gut does not have to work too hard. Gradually, the complexity of the form of the nutrients increases, so the gut will have to start doing more work. Dietary fat is part of the regimen in the form of medium-chain triglycerides (MCT), which do not require emulsification and minimal enzyme activity for digestion. MCT provides valuable calories at a time when weight loss is a problem to solve.

Immediately Following Intestinal Resection Surgery

- Parenteral nutrition is required. The extent of the resection and overall health of the subject will determine the duration of parenteral nutrition.

- Enteral nutrition should begin as soon as possible after surgery.

Oral Diet

- Diet should progress slowly over several weeks or months, depending on the speed of the intestinal adaptation process (which may take up to one year).

- Supplemental tube feedings may be necessary during this time. Optimally, enteral formulas should include nucleotides; glutamine; short-chain fatty acids (butyrate, proprionate, acetate); and fiber. Feedings should begin at 1,500 milliliters per day over several hours and be increased as tolerated.

- Transitional diet from enteral formulas to oral diet should be high in fat (with use of MCT oil) and low in carbohydrate.

As oral diet tolerance improves

- Reduce fat intake to 40 to 50 grams per day with use of MCT oil. Fat intake may be increased for weight gain as tolerated.

- Increase protein intake to 1.5 to 2 g/kg/day.

- Increase calorie intake to 35 to 45 calories/kg/day.

- Foods to avoid (a bland diet may be preferred): caffeine; concentrated sweets; Mannitol, Sorbitol, Xylitol, lactose.

- Avoid high-oxalate foods: beets, celery, chocolate and cocoa, high doses of vitamin C, nuts, peanut butter, rhubarb, spinach, strawberries, sweet potatoes, tea, wheat bran.

- Choose chewable or liquid vitamin and mineral supplements that include calcium, magnesium, zinc, iron, manganese, vitamin C, selenium, potassium, folic acid, B-complex vitamins, and water-miscible forms of vitamins A, D, E, and K.

Figure 8.5 Dietary Recommendations for Short Bowel Syndrome

- Parenteral administration of vitamin B_{12} is likely needed.
- If supplemental medium-chain triglyceride oil is used, divide it into doses of 1 tablespoon and take throughout the day with meals.

Diet and Behavior Modifications
- Eat six to ten small meals daily.
- Consume fluids between meals in small amounts.

Possible Modified Diet-Induced Deficiencies
- Calcium
- Riboflavin
- Vitamins A, D, E, and K

Figure 8.5 *Continued*

Next, the volume of the parenteral feeding is gradually reduced, and enteral feeding takes the front seat. When the person can begin eating food again, the approach is again gradual (see Figure 8.6). Small, frequent meals are helpful, and low fiber can help reduce stool output. For most people, eating food at both extremes of temperature and caffeine increases intestinal motility, which may aggravate diarrhea. A low-fat diet helps control possible steatorrhea, and a low-oxalate diet can help stave off the complication of kidney stones. The MCT supplement can help to add extra calories on the low-fat diet, but this type of fat does not provide the essential fatty acids, linoleic and linolenic. A small amount of vegetable oil (less than a teaspoon) can provide these nutrients.

Because digestive enzymes are in short supply, most people with short bowel syndrome will be lactose intolerant. In avoiding dairy products, the person with short bowel syndrome must remember to supplement nutrients such as calcium and vitamin D, which are plentiful in dairy products. Concentrated sweets may pose problems, partly because of inadequate levels of the enzyme to digest the sugar but also because these foods are hyperosmolar and may contribute to dumping

Breakfast

- 1   hard-boiled egg
- 1   slice toast
- 1   teaspoon margarine
- ½   cup unsweetened applesauce

Snack

- ½   cup calcium-fortified orange juice
- ¾   cup cereal

Snack

- 4   ounces isotonic high-protein liquid supplement

Lunch

- 3   ounces meat loaf
- ½   cup sliced, boiled summer squash
- ½   cup rice pilaf (no nuts)
- ½   cup fruit cocktail (juice packed)

Snack

- ½   cup calcium-fortified juice
- 2   plain bread sticks

Snack

- 4   ounces isotonic high-protein liquid supplement

Dinner

- 3   ounces baked Atlantic salmon
- ½   cup canned carrots
- 1   dinner roll
- 1   teaspoon margarine
- 1   banana

Snack

- ½   cup calcium-fortified juice
- 2   ounces oven-roasted turkey breast
- 1   slice pita bread
- 1   tablespoon low-fat mayonnaise

Calories 1,829; protein 92 g (20%); fat 42 g (24%); carbohydrate 255 g (56%); cholesterol 343 mg; calcium 811 mg; sodium 3,487 mg; fiber 15 g.

Figure 8.6 Sample Menu for Short Bowel Syndrome

syndrome. Other ways to prevent dumping are to drink liquids only between meals and to avoid drinking with meals.

Several medications are useful in treating short bowel syndrome. Cholestyramine can help with diarrhea, but it can also cause constipation, nausea, and vomiting. Other antidiarrheals are often used, and determining the cause of the diarrhea will assist in selecting the best drug. Medications called enzyme replacements supplement the deficient digestive enzymes, and the replacement for a fat-digesting enzyme is particularly useful in short bowel syndrome. One of the problems with this syndrome can be excess gastric acid secretion, so using drugs such as cimetidine and omeprazole reduces acid output. Because of the likelihood of bacterial overgrowth and the development of blind loop, antibiotics become important treatments in short bowel syndrome.

Intestinal adaptation typically takes up to one year after the intestinal surgery. Research on intestinal adaptation has given people with short bowel syndrome hope for relief of the malabsorption and its symptoms. So far, gut enhancers (compounds that accelerate intestinal adaptation) with the most solid evidence behind them are glutamine, nucleotides, and short-chain fatty acids. These gut enhancers benefit the intestine by serving as primary fuel sources for the intestinal cells. Glutamine is the favorite fuel of small intestine cells, whereas colon cells like short-chain fatty acids best. Food, which naturally contains thousands of chemicals, is one of the best gut enhancers, which is why returning to as normal a diet as possible is so important.

Gut Enhancers Glutamine, an amino acid, is widely available in most foods that contain protein and is the amino acid present in the highest levels in blood. The intestinal cells and other rapidly dividing cells use glutamine as their favorite energy source; the liver then takes the two by-products, ammonia and the amino acid alanine, to make urea and glucose. All body cells use glutamine to synthesize new amino acids and proteins. Most people who are healthy do not need to eat foods containing glutamine, because it is a nonessential amino acid, which means that the body can make it. In times of acute physiologic stress, and especially after intestinal resection, however, the dietary supply falls short. Scientists now consider this amino acid conditionally essential, meaning that normally the body does not need to get it from the diet, but that in certain conditions the body cannot keep up with the demand. Research has shown that after intestinal resection, adding glutamine to a parenteral feeding solution promotes intestinal adaptation.[9]

Short-chain fatty acids, which include butyrate, propionate, and acetate, have demonstrated their value in the health of the GI tract in many ways. Researchers have long known that they serve as an important energy source to the cells of the colon; even in healthy people, short-chain fatty acids provide 5 to 10 percent of the total day's energy. After resection, they may provide up to 1,000 calories per day! That figure is even more impressive considering that resection patients need high energy because of malabsorption. Now, new studies are describing the role of short-chain fatty acids as gut enhancers after intestinal resection. The first effect of short-chain fatty acids that helps after resection is their ability to stimulate intestinal growth, which is critical in allowing the remaining intestine to carry on the digestive and absorption functions. In addition, they increase blood flow to the intestine, helping to nourish the cells because blood carries the oxygen and nutrients to body cells. They also appear to stimulate the pancreas to secrete its digestive enzymes and encourage the colon to carry out its functions of water and electrolyte reabsorption. Bacteria in the colon help by cranking out short-chain fatty acids after digesting fiber. To do their magic, though, the bacteria need a good supply of carbohydrate, especially complex carbohdyrates containing fiber. After resection, a high-carbohydrate diet helps to generate short-chain fatty acids and promote adaptation.

Researchers have identified two hormones produced by the body, growth hormone and insulin-like growth factor (IGF-1), that appear to promote intestinal adaptation. Growth hormone stimulates tissue growth, so its usefulness as a gut enhancer is obvious. IGF-1 works in tandem with growth hormone by serving as the direct stimulating agent in coaxing intestinal cells to grow. Glutamine also plays a role by increasing the levels of growth hormone. Researchers also believe that a host of other compounds—including the hormones, gastrin, insulin, cholecystokinin, glucagon, and compounds such as glucose, dietary fiber, and dietary fats—can act as gut enhancers.

Conclusion

■ · · · · · · ■

After this short journey through the center of the body, it would be hard not to stand in awe of the intricate and nifty design of the human gastrointestinal system. From the precision of nutrient absorption to the system's ability to put up with whatever is thrown down it over decades of a lifetime, it is certainly a thing of beauty. Even with the many diseases or conditions that can affect the GI tract, its resilience and ability to adapt is nothing short of miraculous. Another key point about GI diseases and conditions, however, is their potential to affect nutritional status, and therefore the health of a person, profoundly.

If one were to suggest an improvement on the design, however, it would be to make symptoms of each disease unique and unmistakable. Because the GI tract has a limited repertoire of responses to injury and disease, it is easy to mistake one disease for another. Worse yet, many people attribute their symptoms to a "touch of food poisoning" or "touchy digestion." The obvious problem with these typical reactions is that a disease process continues to do damage when left untreated. From a nutritional standpoint, even the simple self-treatment of avoiding suspected foods can deprive the body of essential nutrients.

The connection between nutritional status and overall health is impossible to separate. When a person's nutrient stores and status are low, he or she cannot adequately fend off an attack, whether it comes from an outside invader, such as an infection, or from the body itself, as in inflammatory bowel disease. Likewise, a seemingly simple problem, such as chronic diarrhea, robs a person's nutritional store, making off with the valuables of protein, vitamins, and minerals.

Research has proven that the gastrointestinal system and a person's nutrition, which includes the foods and the nutrients they provide every day and the body's nutrient status, are intimately intertwined. Here's to your continued good digestion, appetite, and health.

Resources

■ · · · · · · ■

General Gastrointestinal Disease

CDC International Travelers Health Line (traveler's diarrhea)
404/332-4555

Digestive Disease National Coalition
507 Capitol Court NE, Suite 200
Washington, DC 20002
202/544-7497

Intestinal Disease Foundation
1323 Forbes Avenue, Suite 200
Pittsburgh, PA 15219
412/261-5888

National Digestive Diseases Information Clearinghouse
Two Information Way
Bethesda, MD 20892-3570
301/654-3810
www.aoa.dhhs.gov/aoa/dir/154.html

Gastritis and Ulcers

888/MY-ULCER
800/NO-ULCER

H. pylori Education Campaign
Division of Bacterial and Mycotic Diseases
National Center for Infectious Diseases
Centers for Disease Control and Prevention
1600 Clifton Road, MS: C09
Atlanta, GA 30333
www.cdc.gov

Gastroesophageal Reflux Disease (GERD)

GERD hotline: 800/478-2876

GERD treatment (endo lumenal gastroplication) hotline: 800/436-7936

www.HeartburnAlliance.org

www.gerd.com

Center for Ulcer Research and Education Foundation
11661 San Vicente Boulevard, Suite 304
Los Angeles, CA 90049
213/825-5091

Inflammatory Bowel Diseases

Crohn's & Colitis Foundation of America
386 Park Avenue South, 17th Floor
New York, NY 10016
800/343-3637
www.ccfa.org

Celiac Disease

American Celiac Society (ACS)
45 Gifford Avenue
Jersey City, NJ 07304
201/432-1207

Ostomy

United Ostomy Association
19772 MacArthur Boulevard, Suite 200
Irvine, CA 92614
800/826-0826; 714/660-8624
E-mail: uoa@deltanet.com
www.uoa.org

Notes

■ . . . . ■

Introduction

1. K. B. Taylor, "Gastrointestinal Disease and Nutritional Status," *Comprehensive Therapy* 12 (1979): 45–77.

Chapter 3

1. S. F. Ahsan, R. J. Meleca, and J. P. Dworkin, "Botulinum Toxin Injection of the Cricopharyngeus Muscle for the Treatment of Dysphagia," *Otolaryngology Head and Neck Surgery* 122(5) (2000): 691–95.

2. T. Arai et al., "Technetium Tin Colloid Test Detecting Symptomless Dysphagia and ACE Inhibitor Prevented Occurrence of Aspiration Pneumonia," *International Journal of Molecular Medicine* 5(6) (2000): 609–10.

3. P. M. Bath, F. I. Bath, and D. G. Smithard, "Interventions for Dysphagia in Acute Stroke," *Cochrane Database of Systematic Reviews* 2 (2000): CD000323.

4. A. Kjellin, et al., "Gastroesophageal Reflux in Obese Patients Is Not Reduced by Weight Reduction," *Scandinavian Journal of Gastroenterology* 31(11) (1996): 1047–51.

5. A. Kjellin, et al., "Gastroesophageal Reflux," edited by S. Escott-Stump and L. Mahan. In *Krause's Food, Nutrition, and Diet Therapy*, 10th ed., Philadelphia: Saunders, 2000.

6. C. E. Ruhl and J. E. Everhart, "Overweight, But Not High Dietary Fat Intake, Increases Risk of Gastroesophageal Reflux Disease Hospitalization: The NHANES I Epidemiologic Followup Study." First National Health and Nutrition Examination Survey, *Annals of Epidemiology* 9(7) (October 1999): 424–35.

7. L. J. WILSON, W. MA, and B. I. HIRSCHOWITZ, "Association of Obesity with Hiatal Hernia and Esophagitis," *American Journal of Gastroenterology* 94(10) (October 1999): 2840–44.

8. J. P. GISBERT, J. M. PAJARES, and C. LOSA, "*Helicobacter pylori* and Gastroesophageal Reflux Disease: Friends or Foes," *Hepato-Gastroenterology* 34 (7): (July 1999) 1023–29.

9. D. McNAMARA and C. O'MORAIN, "Gastroesophageal Reflux Disease and *Helicobacter pylori*: An Intricate Relation," *Gut* 45(suppl. 1) (1999): 113–17.

10. GISBERT, PAJARES, and LOSA, "*Heliobacter pylori* and Gastroesophageal Reflux Disease."

11. K. E. McCOLL, "The Role of *Heliobacter pylori* Infection in GERD," *Scandinavian Journal of Gastroenterology* 35(1) (2000): 111–12.

12. G. HOLTMANN, C. CAIN, and P. MALFERTHEINER, "Gastric *Helicobacter pylori* Infection Accelerates Healing of Reflux Esophagitis During Treatment with the Proton Pump Inhibitor Pantoprazole," *Gastroenterology* 117 (1999): 11–16.

13. McNAMARA and O'MORAIN, "Gastroesophageal Reflux Disease."

14. "The 1996 Canadian Outook on GERD, Consensus Conference, Ottawa, Ontario, June 1996," *Canadian Journal of Gastroenterology* (11 Suppl B) (September 1997): B–112B.

15. J. P. GALMICHE, "Gastro-Oesophageal Reflux: Does It Matter What You Eat?" *Gut* 42 (1998): 318–19.

16. R. PENAGINI, M. MANGANO, and P. A. BIANCHI, "Effect of Increasing the Fat Content But Not the Energy Load of a Meal on Gastro-Oesophageal Reflux and Lower Oesophageal Sphincter Motor Function," *Gut* 42 (1998): 330–33.

17. R. H. HOLLOWAY ET AL., "Effect of Intraduodenal Fat on Lower Oesophageal Sphincter Function and Gastro-Oesophageal Reflux," *Gut* 40 (1997): 449–53.

18. PENAGINI, MANGANO, and BIANCHI, "Effect of Increasing the Fat Content."

19. Megan Christensen, June 20, 2000. *Detroit Free Press.*

20. *Detroit Free Press,* June 20, 2000.

21. J. DENT, "The Hiatus Hernia Slides Back into Prominence," *Gut* 44 (1999): 449–50.

22. P. J. KAHRILAS ET AL., "The Effect of Hiatus Hernia on Gastroesophageal Junction Pressure," *Gut* 44 (1999): 476–82.

23. A. D. JENKINSON, S.M. SCOTT, and S.S. KADIRKAMANATHAN, "Vector Manometry and LOS Dynamics," *Gut* 46 (2000): 740.

24. M. FEIN ET AL., "Role of the Lower Esophageal Sphincter and Hiatal Hernia in the Pathogenesis of Gastroesophageal Reflux Disease," *Journal of Gastrointestinal Surgery* 3(4) (July–August 1999): 405–10; P. J. KAHRILAS ET AL., "Increased Frequency of Transient Lower Esophageal Sphincter Relaxation Induced by Gastric Distention in Reflux Patients with Hiatal Hernia," *Gastroenterology* 118 (2000): 688–95.

25. J. DENT, "The Hiatus Hernia."

26. I. J. CARRE ET AL., "Familial Hiatal Hernia in a Large Five Generation Family Confirming True Autosomal Dominant Inheritance," *Gut* 45 (1999): 649–52.

27. S. M. BAGLAJ and H. R. NOBLETT, "Paraesophageal Hernia in Children: Familial Occurrence and Review of the Literature," *Pediatric Surgery International* 15(2) (1999): 85–7.

28. I. J. CARRE ET AL., "Familial Hiatal Hernia."

Chapter 4

1. B. J. MARSHALL, "*Helicobacter pylori*: A Primer for 1994," *Gastroenterology* 1(4) (1993): 241–47.

2. A. TOYONAGA ET AL., "Epidemiological Study on Food Intake and *Helicobacter pylori* Infection," *Kurume Medical Journal* 47(1) (2000): 25–30.

3. U. BLECKER, D. I. MEHTA, and B. D. GOLD, "Pediatric Gastritis and Peptic Ulcer Disease," *Indian Journal of Pediatrics* 66(5) (September–October 1999): 725–33.

4. L. BENINI ET AL., "Gastric Emptying of Solids is Markedly Delayed When Meals Are Fried," *Digestive Diseases and Science* 39(11) (1994): 2288–94.

5. W. H. ALDOORI ET AL., "Prospective Study of Diet and the Risk of Duodenal Ulcer in Men," *American Journal of Epidemiology*, 145(1) (January 1 1997): 42–50

6. G. IDDAN ET AL., "Wireless Capsule Endoscopy," *Nature* 405 (May 25 2000): 417.

7. C. LA VECCHIA, A. DECARLI, and R. PAGANO, "Vegetable Consumption and Risk of Chronic Disease," *Epidemiology* 9(2) (March 1998): 208–10.

8. J. W. Lampe, "Health Effects of Vegetables and Fruit: Assessing Mechanisms of Action in Human Experimental Studies," *American Journal of Clinical Nutrition* 70(3 Suppl) (September 1999): 475S–90S.

9. M. K.SERDULA, ET AL., "The Association Between Fruit and Vegetable Intake and Chronic Disease Risk Factors," *Epidemiology* 7(2) (March 1996): 161–65.

10. S. LEVENSTEIN, "Stress and Peptic Ulcer: Life Beyond *Helicobacter*," *British Medical Journal* 316 (1998): 538–41.

11. R. J. PLAYFORD ET AL., "Bovine Colostrum Is a Health Food Supplement Which Prevents NSAID Induced Gut Damage," *Gut* 44 (1999): 653–58.

12. V. MANJARI and U. N. DAS, "Effect of Polyunsaturated Fatty Acids on Dexamethasone-Induced Gastric Mucosal Damage," *Prostaglandins Leukotrienes, and Essential Fatty Acids* 62(2) (February 2000): 85–96.

13. ———"Effect of Polyunsaturated Fatty Acids;" U. N. DAS, "Hypothesis: Cis-Unsaturated Fatty Acids as Potential Anti-Peptic Ulcer Drugs," *Prostaglandins Leukotrienes Essential Fatty Acids* 58(5) (May 1998): 377–80. (Abstract)

14. MANJARI and DAS, "Effect of Polyunsaturated Fatty Acids."

15. DAS, "Hypothesis."

16. W. H. ALDOORI ET AL., "A Prospective Study of Alcohol, Smoking, Caffeine, and the Risk of Duodenal Ulcer in Men," *Epidemiology* (4) (July 1997): 420–24.

Chapter 5

1. A. STROCCHI and M. D. LEVITT, "Intestinal Gas." In *Gastrointestinal and Liver Disease*, edited by M. Feldman, M. H. Sleisenger, and B. F. Scharshcmidt, 6th ed. Philadelphia: Saunders, 1998.

2. B. A. PRIBILA ET AL., "Improved Lactose Digestion and Tolerance Among African-American Adolescent Girls Fed a Dairy-Rich Diet, *Journal of the American Dietetic Association* 100(5) (May 2000): 524–28.

3. PRIBILA ET AL., "Improved Lactose Digestion and Tolerance."

4. A. CARROCCIO ET AL., "Lactose Intolerance and Self-Reported Milk Intolerance: Relationship with Lactose Maldigestion and Nutrient Intake, Lactase Deficiency Study Group," *Journal of the American College of Nutrition* 17 (6) (December 1998): 631–36.

5. Nutrition News Focus, "*Misconceptions About Milk*," www.nutrition-newsfocus.com, June 4, 2000.

6. Nutrition News Focus, "*Misconceptions About Milk*," January 20, 1999.

7. U. TEURI, H. VAPAATALO, and R. KORPELA, "Fructooligosaccharides and

Lactulose Cause More Symptoms in Lactose Maldigesters and Subjects with Pseudohypolactasia Than in Control Lactose Digesters," *American Journal of Clinical Nutrition* 69(5) (1999): 973–79.

8. ———, "Fructooligosaccharides and Lactulose"; S. Mishkin, "Dairy Products for the Lactose Intolerant," *Nutrition and the M.D.* 26(1) (2000): 5–6.

Chapter 6

1. L. KOHLER, S. SAUERLAND, and E. NEUGEBAUER, "Diagnosis and Treatment of Diverticular Disease: Results of a Consensus Development Conference, the Scientific Committee of the European Association for Endoscopic Surgery," *Surgical Endoscopy* 13(4) (1999): 430–36.

2. W. H. ALDOORI ET AL., "A Prospective Study of Dietary Fiber Types and Symptomatic Diverticular Disease in Men," *Journal of Nutrition* 128(4) (1998): 714–19.

3. M. E. SHILS ET AL., *Modern Nutrition in Health and Disease,* 9th ed. (Baltimore: Williams and Wilkins, 1999).

4. M. V. KENNEDY and E. J. ZARLING, "Answers to 10 Key Questions on Diverticular Disease of the Colon," *Comprehensive Therapy* 24(8) (1998): 364–69.

5. D. A. DROSSMAN ET AL., "Irritable Bowel Syndrome: A Technical Review for Practice Guideline Development," *Gastroenterology* 112 (1997): 2120.

6. W. G. PATERSON ET AL., "Recommendations for the Management of Irritable Bowel Syndrome in Family Practice, IBS Consensus Conference Participants," *Canadian Medical Association Journal* 161(2) (July 27 1999): 154–60.

7. *Merck Manual,* 17th ed. (Whitehouse Station, N. J.: Merck Research Laboratories, 1999).

8. PATERSON ET AL., "Recommendations."

9. M. H. PITTLER and E. ERNST, "Peppermint Oil for Irritable Bowel Syndrome: A Critical Review and Metaanalysis," *American Journal of Gastroenterology* 93 (1998): 1131–35.

10. *Merck Manual,* 17th ed.

11. PITTLER and ERNST, "Peppermint Oil for Irritable Bowel Syndrome."

12. T. H. VESA ET AL., "Role of Irritable Bowel Syndrome in Subjective Lactose Intolerance. *American Journal of Clinical Nutrition* 67 (1998): 710–15.

13. ———., "Role of Irritable Bowel Syndrome;" R. MASCOLO, and J. R. SALTZMAN, "Lactose Intolerance and Irritable Bowel Syndrome," *Nutrition Reviews* 56(10) (October 1998): 306–8.

14. A. D. SHAW and G. J. DAVIES, "Lactose Intolerance: Problems in Diag-

nosis and Treatment," *Journal of Clinical Gastroenterology* 28(3) (April 1999): 208–16.

15. T. E. GALOVSKI and E. B. BLANCHARD, "The Treatment of Irritable Bowel Syndrome with Hypnotherapy," *Applied Psychophysiology and Biofeedback* 23(4) (December 1998): 219–32.

16. *Detroit Free Press*, May 25, 1999, Medical News Briefs.

17. M. VIDAKOVIC-VUKIC, "Hypnotherapy in the Treatment of Irritable Bowel Syndrome: Methods and Results in Amsterdam," *Scandinavian Journal of Gastroenterology* 34(230) (1999): 49–51.

18. G. SPELLET, "Nutritional Management of Common Gastrointestinal Problems," *Nurse Practitioner Forum* 5 (1994): 24.

Chapter 7

1. S. C. BISCHOFF ET AL., "Prevalence of Adverse Reactions to Food in Patients with Gastrointestinal Disease, *Allergy* 51 (1996): 811.

2. R. SHODA ET AL., "Epidemiologic Analysis of Crohn's Disease in Japan: Increased Dietary Intake of n-6 Polyunsaturated Fatty Acids and Animal Protein Relates to Increased Incidence of Crohn's Disease in Japan," *American Journal of Clinical Nutrition* 63 (1996): 741.

3. F. A. EL-ZAATARI ET AL., "Characterization of Mycobacterium Paratuberculosis p36 Antigen and Its Seroreactivities in Crohn's Disease," *Current Issues in Intestinal Microbiology* 39(2) (1999): 115–19.

4. S. VERMA ET AL., "Polymeric Versus Elemental Diet as Primary Treatment in Active Crohn's Disease: A Randomized, Double-Blind Trial." *American Journal of Gastroenterology* 95(3) (2000): 735–39.

5. H. IKEUCHI ET AL., "Effects of Elemental Diet on Surgical Treatment in Crohn's Disease." *Hepato-Gastroenterology* 47(32) (2000): 390–92.

6. B. G. FEAGAN ET AL., "A Comparison of Methotrexate with Placebo for the Maintenance of Remission in Crohn's Disease, North American Crohn's Study Group Investigators," *New England Journal of Medicine* 342(22) (June 1, 2000):1627–32.

7. A. E. SLONIM ET AL., "A Preliminary Study of Growth Hormone Therapy for Crohn's Disease," *New England Journal of Medicine* 342(22) (June 1, 2000): 1633–37.

8. B. J. GEERLING ET AL., "The Relation Between Antioxidant Status and Alterations in Fatty Acid Profile in Patients with Crohn's Disease and Controls," *Scandinavian Journal of Gastroenterology* 34 (1999): 1108–16.

9. L. A. DIELEMAN and W. D. HEIZER, "Nutritional Issues in Inflammatory Bowel Disease," *Gastroenterology Clinics of North America* 27(2) (June 1998): 435–51.

10. B. J. GEERLING, ET AL., "Fat Intake and Fatty Acid Profile in Plasma Phospholipids and Adipose Tissue in Patients with Crohn's Disease, Compared with Controls," *Journal of Gastroenterology* 94(2) (February 1999): 410–16.

11. S. BJORCK ET AL., "Food-Induced Stimulation of the Anti-secretory Factor Can Improve Symptoms in Human Inflammatory Bowel Disease: A Study of a Concept," *Gut* 46(6) (2000): 743–45.

12. G. D'ARGENIO and G. MAZZACCA, "Short-Chain Fatty Acid in the Human Colon: Relation to Inflammatory Bowel Diseases and Colon Cancer," *Advanced Experiments in Medical Biology* 472 (1999): 149–58.

13. J. A. Murray, "The Widening Spectrum of Celiac Disease," *American Journal of Clinical Nutrition* 69(3) (1999): 354–65.

14. J. L. SHAKER ET AL., "Hypocalcemia and Skeletal Disease as Presenting Features of Celiac Disease," *Archives of Internal Medicine* 157(9) (1997): 1013–16.

15. M. T. BARDELLA ET AL., "Increased Prevalence of Celiac Disease in Patients with Dyspepsia," *Archives of Internal Medicine* 160(10) (May 22, 2000): 1489–91.

16. T. Thompson, "Thiamin, Riboflavin, and Niacin Contents of the Gluten-Free Diet: Is There Cause for Concern?" *Journal of the American Dietetic Association* 99(7) (1999): 858–62.

17. ———, "Do Oats Belong in a Gluten-Free Diet?" *Journal of the American Dietetic Association* 97(12) (1997): 1413–16.

18. THOMPSON, "Do Oats Belong"; E. K. JANATUINEN ET AL., "Lack of Cellular and Humoral Immunological Responses to Oats in Adults with Coeliac Disease," *Gut* 46(3) (March 2000): 327–31; MURRAY, "The Widening Spectrum"; THOMPSON, "Questionable Foods and the Gluten-Free Diet: Survey of Current Recommendations," *Journal of the American Dietetic Association* 100(4) (2000): 463–65.

19. JANATUINEN ET AL., "Lack of Cellular and Humoral Immunological Responses."

20. MURRAY, "The Widening Spectrum of Celiac Disease."

21. THOMPSON, "Questionable Foods."

22. THOMPSON, "Do Oats Belong. "

23. THOMPSON, "Questionable Foods."

24. THOMPSON, "Do Oats Belong."

Chapter 8

1. N. S. GOLDSTEIN ET AL., "Crohn's-Like Complications in Patients with Ulcerative Colitis After Total Proctocolectomy and Ileal Pouch-Anal Anastomosis," *American Journal of Surgical Pathology* 21 (1997): 1343.

2. L. A. Dieleman and W. D. Heizer, "Nutritional Issues in Inflammatory Bowel Disease," *Gastroenterology Clinics of North America* 27(2) (June 1998): 435–51.

3. I. NORDGAARD, B. S. HANSEN, and P. B. MORTENSEN, "Importance of Colonic Support for Energy Absorption as Small Bowel Failure Proceeds," *American Journal of Clinical Nutrition* 64 (1996): 222–31.

4. J. BUENO ET AL., "Factors Impacting the Survival of Children with Intestinal Failure Referred for Intestinal Transplantation," *Pediatric Surgery* 34(1) (January 1999): 27–33.

5. H. J. SILVER and V. H. CASTELLANOS, "Nutritional Complications and Management of Intestinal Transplant," *Journal of the American Dietetic Association* 100(6) (2000): 680–89.

6. S. MISHKIN, "Growth Factors and Short Bowel Syndrome," *Nutrition and the M.D.* 26(1) (2000): 5.

7. J.M.B. NIGHTINGALE, "Management of Patients with a Short Bowel," *Nutrition* 15(1999): 633–37.

8. G. SAVY, "Everything You Ever Wanted to Know About Glutamine," *Today's Dietitian* (September 1999): 52–55.

9. T. R. ZIEGLER ET AL., "Glutamine and the Gastrointestinal Tract," *Current Opinion in Clinical Nutrition and Metabolic Care* 3(5) (September 2000): 355–62.

Glossary

■ · · · · · · · ■

absorption The process by which the intestinal cells assimilate digested nutrients. The intestinal cells line the surface of finger-like projections, called *villi*, which in turn line folds of tissue within the intestine. Once absorbed into the intestinal cell, a nutrient can pass either into the bloodstream through capillaries or into the lymphatic system. Water-soluble nutrients can enter the bloodstream, but fat-soluble nutrients (vitamins A, D, E, and K) go through the lymphatic system. Virtually all nutrients are absorbed in the small intestine, with most absorption occurring in the upper portions of the small intestine.

achalasia A neuromuscular disorder that causes difficulty in swallowing because of problems with abnormal esophageal contractions and inability of the lower esophageal sphincter to open as swallowed food nears. Eating is painful, because the esophagus becomes distended. Diet therapy consists of small, frequent meals; avoidance of difficult-to-swallow, acidic, or spicy foods that could damage the irritated esophageal tissue; and a bland diet if it is better tolerated. Drugs can allow the lower esophageal sphincter (LES) to relax and open. Surgical treatment involves weakening the lower esophageal sphincter, but that may result in reflux.

achlorhydria A low level of gastric acidity, which is common in the elderly and among people who have had stomach surgery.

The low acidity leads to improper absorption of iron and vitamin B$_{12}$, which require an acidic environment for absorption.
Also, the first step in protein digestion is uncoiling of the mole-
cule by an acid environment.

albumin The main blood protein, which is used as one parameter
in assessment of nutritional status. The normal level of albumin
in blood is 3.5 to 5.0 grams. Low levels of blood albumin indicate
protein depletion, although the level of albumin is also affected
by hydration status. If a person is dehydrated, albumin will be
falsely high; if a person is overhydrated albumin will be falsely
low. The liver makes albumin, so when that organ is not functioning properly, blood albumin levels may be low. In the blood,
albumin has several functions, including maintaining fluid
balance and transporting nutrients.

alimentary tract Another term for the gastrointestinal tract, which
includes the mouth, esophagus, stomach, small intestine, and
large intestine.

amino acid The smallest unit that makes up the backbone of a
protein. Humans need nine amino acids, called *essential amino
acids*, to make other amino acids and finally proteins.
Protein is the building material for body tissues, which make
up organs, muscle, blood cells, and enzymes. The nine
essential amino acids are histadine, isoleucine, leucine, lysine,
methionine, phenylalanine, threonine, tryptophan, and valine.
In general, foods derived from animals, such as meat and
dairy products, have a higher proportion of the essential amino
acids compared to plant-based foods. The higher the proportion
of the nine essential amino acids in a food, the higher the
quality of the protein.

anemia (iron deficiency) Deficiency of iron, characterized
by small, pale red blood cells. Symptoms include pale skin,
weakness, lethargy, dizziness, and lack of appetite. Iron defi-

ciency anemia may be caused by poor dietary intake, chronic blood loss as in GI bleeding, and increased need. Iron supplementation, along with a diet high in iron, can usually reverse the problem. If blood iron is severely low, however, a blood transfusion may be necessary.

antacid A medication that lowers the acidity level of the stomach by buffering acid. Antacids consist of inorganic salts that dissolve in acid and release negatively charged particles that neutralize hydrochloric acid in the stomach. They are a useful treatment in many upper GI disorders, but they may cause side effects. Nutritional side effects include reduction in absorption of iron, vitamin B_{12}, and vitamin A; they also deplete phosphorus levels and destroy thiamin. GI side effects include bloating, cramping, and constipation.

antibiotic An antimicrobial agent used to treat infections or reduce the number of microbes. In GI diseases, antibiotics are the first-line treatment for eradicating *H. pylori*, the bacteria that causes gastritis and peptic ulcer disease. Antibiotics are also used to destroy the overgrowth of bacteria, which arise in blind loop syndrome. Antibiotics used for other conditions can wipe out friendly bacteria that inhabit the colon and serve several useful purposes. In this case, diet can be changed to encourage the reintroduction of bacteria in the colon. Various antibiotics have potentially serious side effects, including GI effects such as nausea, diarrhea, and interference with absorption or use of specific nutrients.

anticholinergics Drugs that interfere with the receptors for acetylcholine, a compound that transmits nerve impulses of the parasympathetic nervous system. These drugs are useful in the treatment of certain GI problems because they reduce intestinal muscle spasms, decrease GI secretions, and relax the lower esophageal sphincter, allowing it to open.

antiulcer agents A group of drugs that allow ulcers to heal either
  by interference with gastric acid secretion (also called *anti-
  secretory agents*), or by formation of a protective mucosal barrier.
  These drugs include cimetadine (Tagamet), famotidine
  (Pepcid), lansoprazole (Prevacid), nizatidine (Axid), omeprazole
  (Prilosec), and ranitidine (Zantac).

atrophic gastritis A disease thought to be caused by the attack of
  antibodies in the stomach's lining in which all layers of the
  stomach become inflamed. The result is thinning of the lining
  and loss of acid and enzyme-producing cells. It is common
  among elderly people and in people who have had partial
  gastrectomy. Atrophic gastritis can cause pernicious anemia, the
  deficiency of B_{12}, and iron-deficiency anemia because of the low
  acidity level in the stomach.

autoimmune disorder A disorder in which the body's immune
  system attacks its own tissues. Normally, a foreign invader,
  an antigen, enters the body, and the immune system responds
  by release of antibodies to destroy the antigen. In autoimmunity,
  the attack is unleashed on the body's own cells. GI disease
  examples include the inflammatory bowel diseases, ulcerative
  colitis, and Crohn's disease. In these diseases, inflammation
  occurs in various layers of the intestine because of immune
  response–induced release of inflammatory compounds. Other
  non-GI autoimmune diseases include multiple sclerosis,
  arthritis, systemic lupus erythematosus, and scleroderma.
  Scientists are still not sure what triggers the immune response,
  but typical treatment includes the use of corticosteroids,
  powerful immunosuppressant agents.

Barnett continent ileostomy (BCI) A procedure done after intestinal resections that creates an internal reservoir for stool,
  making an external appliance unnecessary. It is not recommended in cases of resections due to Crohn's disease, because
  the disease can be expected to strike the small intestine again.

bezoar (phytobezoar) A solid ball of hair or fruit and vegetable fiber that forms in the stomach. One of the most common constituents is the fiber from citrus fruits, such as oranges and tangerines. Bezoars cause an obstruction and interfere with normal GI function and motility, and surgery is required for their removal. In some societies, especially the Far East, bezoars are used in the treatment of certain diseases and are thought to possess mystical properties.

bile, bile acids, bile salts A fluid that the liver synthesizes and releases to the gallbladder that allows emulsification of dietary fat so that it can be digested and absorbed. The gallbladder stores and concentrates bile and then ejects the liquid into the small intestine when fat is present in the duodenum. Bile also activates lipases, fat-digesting enzymes from the pancreas. Bile contains bile salts, bile acids, cholesterol, and lecithin. After it serves its function in the upper portion of the small intestine, it is reabsorbed by the terminal ileum and recirculated back to the liver. Problems in either the terminal ileum (as with Crohn's disease and celiac disease), the liver, the gallbladder, or the ducts connecting the gallbladder to the small intestine result in fat malabsorption.

bland diet A diet used to treat GI diseases such as peptic ulcer disease, esophagitis, or used as a transitional diet. It most typically eliminates known gastric irritants or substances that increase gastric secretion. Some hospitals also eliminate fried foods in addition to gastric irritants. The diet should be individualized and only those foods or substances that provoke an adverse GI response should be eliminated.

blind loop A stagnant segment of the intestine that encourages bacteria overgrowth. Blind loop can be the result of intestinal surgery, obstruction, strictures, or adhesions. The major consequence is fat malabsorption, which causes steatorrhea, weight loss, vitamin B_{12} deficiency, kidney stones, gallstones, and bone disease. The condition is treated with antibiotics, a low-fat and low-oxalate diet, nutritional supplements to counter nutrient losses, and sometimes surgery to repair the blind loop.

bolus In tube feeding, the administration of an entire amount of formula feeding at one time. Other options are to use a pump to infuse the tube feeding continuously over a twenty-four-hour period, or to infuse a specific amount on an intermittent basis. The advantages of a bolus feeding is that it more closely simulates normal eating, relative to intestinal secretion. The major disadvantage is that it may not be well-tolerated. This method of tube feeding delivery is usually used in a stable person who has been receiving tube feedings over an extended period of time.

borborygmos An audible sound coming from the abdomen caused by intestinal hyperactivity or peristalsis. The sound can be a rumbling, gurgling, or tinkling noise. A physician can hear the sound when using a stethoscope pressed against a person's abdomen.

bowel resection See *resection, bowel*

bulk-forming agent, bulking agent Laxatives containing fiber from various plant products; the indigestible part of carbohydrate that is not broken down by enzymes in the human GI tract. These laxatives usually contain methylcellulose or psyllium seed. The fiber attracts water and softens the stool, increasing its size, which promotes easier bowel movements. When taking this type of laxative, it is important to drink extra fluid; if not, the laxative is ineffective. Bulk-forming agents can cause GI distress, including cramping, bloating, and diarrhea.

calcium An essential mineral needed for bone tissue, blood clotting, nerve transmission, and muscle contraction. Inadequate calcium intake can contribute to bone disorders such as osteomalacia and osteoporosis. GI disorders that cause fat malabsorption promote the loss of calcium into the feces, and the result can be bone disorders. Calcium is also a constituent of certain antacids used in treating upper GI disorders. Some antacids (those containing aluminum) can bind calcium and cause deficiency. Saline laxatives (milk of magnesia) can also interfere with calcium absorption. People with lactose intolerance who avoid dairy products will typically not get the recommended dietary level of calcium and may need a supplement.

carbohydrate malabsorption The digestion and absorption of carbohydrate from food requires certain intestinal enzymes. When a person's enzyme level is inadequate, the carbohydrate will not be digested. Instead, it will pass into the colon where bacteria, which possess enzymes to degrade the compounds, ferment the nutrient, causing diarrhea and other GI problems. In addition, as an intact carbohydrate enters the colon, an osmotic shift of fluid enters the intestine, causing bloating, cramping, gas, and diarrhea. The most common malabsorption is lactase deficiency, followed by sucrase deficiency.

casein The primary protein in dairy products. When the casein in milk comes into contact with the enzyme rennin, in the presence of calcium, it forms milk curd and leaves behind a watery substance called *whey*.

cathartic A substance that promotes evacuation of the bowel by stimulating peristalsis. Other terms that relate to the potency of their actions include laxative, purgative, and drastics. Cathartics have different modes of action, with saline cathartics causing the intestine to fill with fluid by osmotic force and irritating compounds that stimulate peristalsis by actively irritating the intestinal membrane. Bulk-forming cathartics attract water, increase stool size, and soften the stool to stimulate peristalsis. Stool softeners attract water and soften the stool, making it is easier to pass.

celiac disease (celiac sprue, nontropical sprue, gluten-sensitive
    enteropathy, gluten-induced enteropathy) A hereditary disease
    in which there is an intolerance to gliadin and related compounds,
    a fraction of the protein gluten. With celiac disease, when gluten
    is eaten, the small intestinal membrane becomes damaged, caus-
    ing malabsorption of nutrients, weight loss, and GI symptoms.
    Researchers recently discovered that other health problems,
    including bone disease and sterility, may develop before the
    person even experiences GI symptoms. The treatment is a diet
    devoid of gluten, which is contained primarily in wheat, oats,
    rye, and barley. Most people with celiac disease respond well to
    a gluten-free diet, but others may have a severe case and will
    require surgery.

cellulose The fibrous part of a plant that gives it support and
    structure. Humans do not have the enzymes necessary to break
    down cellulose, so it's a form of fiber in the diet.

cholecystokinin A hormone secreted by the intestinal cells in
    response to the presence of fat in the small intestine. It causes the
    gallbladder to contract and eject bile through the common bile
    duct and into the duodenum.

chylomicron A lipoprotein particle made and released by the
    intestinal cells to carry absorbed dietary fat. Chylomicrons trans-
    port fat first through the lymphatic system and then into the
    bloodstream to tissues throughout the body. After eating a meal
    containing fat, it takes up to twelve hours for chylomicrons to be
    cleared from the blood.

chyme A pastelike substance, the partially digested and liquefied
    contents of the stomach, that enters the small intestine in small
    amounts throughout the process of digestion.

cimetadine An antiulcer drug that reduces gastric acid secretion,
    thereby allowing an ulcerated area to heal. Some of its potential
    side effects include dizziness, rash, diarrhea, and confusion
    (this is more common in an elderly person taking high doses).

coffee ground emesis (coffee ground vomitus) Vomit that contains digested blood and resembles coffee grinds. It indicates slow bleeding in the upper GI tract.

colectomy Removal of either the entire colon or a portion of it. If the rectum and anus are removed, a stoma will be created through which waste is excreted.

colitis Inflammation of the large intestine. A common cause is inflammatory bowel disease (ulcerative colitis or Crohn's disease).

colon The large intestine, which includes the cecum, ascending colon, transverse colon, descending colon, sigmoid colon, and rectum. The colon secretes mucus, and its functions are to absorb water and electrolytes from the feces. Bacteria normally inhabit the large intestine and promote the health of the organ by digesting dietary fiber and producing short-chain fatty acids, which serve as fuel for the colonic cells and produce vitamin K.

colonoscopy A procedure in which a flexible fiber-optic tube (endoscope) is pushed through the anus into the length of the colon. The scope allows visualization of the colonic mucosa and also provide a means for obtaining biopsies and performing treatments. Before a colonoscopy, the patient fasts for twelve hours, and ingests a cathartic agent or does an enema to cleanse the bowel prior to the procedure. During the procedure, which lasts up to ninety minutes, the patient is sedated. The results can show the presence of obstructions, strictures, inflammatory bowel disease, diverticula, and lesions.

colostomy Intestinal surgery that involves removing a portion of the intestine and creating a stoma through which waste will be excreted. Unless a special internal reservoir is created, the patient will have to wear an appliance over the stoma into which the stool is excreted.

constipation A change in bowel habits that involves a reduced number or size of stool, difficult-to-pass stool, or the inability to have the normal number of bowel movements in a week. Normal bowel movements vary from one individual to another, although fewer than three bowel movements in one week is considered a state of constipation. After any serious disorders have been ruled out, treatment generally focuses on establishing regular bowel habits, increasing fiber and fluid intake, and encouraging regular physical activity. If after trying the previous recommendations laxatives are prescribed, the person should start with either stool softeners or bulking-forming agents. Some side effects can include nausea, bloating, gas, and diarrhea.

Crohn's disease A form of inflammatory bowel disease in which all layers of the intestine become inflamed and bleed. The disease generally strikes the small intestine, especially the ileum, with colon involvement, but it can occur anywhere along the entire length of the GI tract. Crohn's disease, like ulcerative colitis, is characterized by flare-ups and remissions. Symptoms include severe diarrhea, steatorrhea, and abdominal pain. During flare-ups, a person may require hospitalization. Treatment consists of corticosteroids to counter inflammation and an elemental enteral feeding, if tolerated. If the flare-up is severe, the person may require parenteral nutrition. Because of small intestine involvement, many nutrients are not absorbed, making malnutrition possible. Complications can include fistula, obstruction, strictures, and adhesions. Ultimately, surgery may be needed to remove diseased portions of the intestine.

Curling's ulcer A type of stress ulcer that arises after serious burns. Curling's ulcers typically develop in the duodenum and are deep erosions that often produce severe bleeding. The patient is usually fed parenterally until an oral diet is possible.

diarrhea A change in bowel movements that is either more fluid in consistency or in frequency. The different types of diarrhea include osmotic diarrhea, secretory diarrhea, changes in motility or transit time, and iatrogenic diarrhea. Osmotic diarrhea is caused by the presence of osmotically active particles in the intestine, such as undigested lactose or an unabsorbable salt. Secretory diarrhea is caused by a disease process that increases the secretion of water into the intestine. Changes in motility and transit time can be caused by disease or medications. Iatrogenic diarrhea is caused by a medication or other treatment.

digestion The process by which food is broken down into units that the intestinal cells can absorb. It involves several organs and compounds, such as digestive enzymes, bile, and gastric acid. Digestion begins in the mouth with chewing food into smaller pieces, adding liquid and enzymes from saliva. As the chewed food moves from the esophagus into the stomach, the stomach muscles mechanically digest food by grinding it to a pastelike consistency (food is called *chyme* at this point). Stomach acid helps uncoil proteins so digestive enzymes can attack the bonds and degrade the large molecules. Next, the chyme moves into the first part of the small intestine, the duodenum, where its presence stimulates secretion of hormones and digestive enzymes from the small intestine cells to further break down the chyme. Bile from the gallbladder emulsifies fat so that fat-digesting enzymes can break down fat. As nutrients are digested into the form that can be absorbed, they enter the small intestine cells and into circulation.

diphenoxylate An antidiarrheal medication prescribed to treat diarrhea not caused by infection. Side effects include nausea, abdominal discomfort, intestinal obstruction, and skin rash.

diverticular disease The presence of small pockets in the intestine, usually in the sigmoid colon, that can become inflamed and infected. These pockets are thought to be caused by high pressure inside the colon, and weakening of the colonic muscles. A low-fiber diet, stress, and straining during bowel movements may all contribute to the disease. Diverticulosis is the presence of the pockets and is usually asymptomatic, whereas diverticulitis involves trapped feces within the pocket, causing inflammation and infection. Treatment in the flare-up phase is antibiotics, no food until the inflammation resolves, and fluid and electrolyte replacement. As the flare-up subsides, treatment consists of a low-fiber diet for about four weeks and then progresses to a high-fiber diet, avoiding foods that contain small seeds.

dumping syndrome The movement of gastric contents into the small intestine quickly, causing nausea, vomiting, abdominal pain, diarrhea, and dizziness. It can include a second phase in which similar symptoms occur but are due to hypoglycemia from overexcretion of insulin to balance the fast absorption of glucose. Dumping syndrome is a problem for people who have had part or all of the stomach removed; sometimes it is also a problem with intestinal resections. Dietary treatment includes eating small frequent meals; avoiding temperature extremes in foods; drinking beverages between meals; avoiding caffeine; emphasizing higher protein, moderate fat, and moderate to low carbohydrate; and avoiding concentrated sweets.

duodenal ulcer A form of peptic ulcer disease (PUD) in which the erosions occur in the duodenum. This type of PUD usually involves excessive acid secretion, but the cause in most cases is thought to be a bacteria, *H. pylori*. Treatment includes antibiotics to eradicate the infection if present, antacids, antiulcer drugs, and a diet as tolerated, usually avoiding alcohol and both regular and decaffeinated coffee. Some people prefer to follow a bland diet, which excludes gastric irritants such as pepper.

duodenum The first segment of the small intestine, which is about 10 inches long. The common bile duct enters the duodenum and connects the secretions of the pancreas, liver, and gallbladder. The duodenum releases enzymes and hormones that promote the digestive process. It is the site of absorption for vitamin A, thiamin, iron, calcium, fatty acids, glycerol, amino acids, and monosaccharides.

dyspepsia The medical term for indigestion. It can encompass any of the typical GI symptoms, including nausea, vomiting, abdominal distention, gas, and belching.

dysphagia Difficulty swallowing. It can be of unknown causes, but common reasons include stroke, aging, diseases that affect the nervous system, and the aftereffects of having a nasogastric feeding tube. The major complication is aspiration of food into the lungs with the subsequent development of pneumonia. The dietary approach is to individualize the diet, because the ideal consistency varies for each person. Many people with dysphagia have more success with thickened liquids (commercial products can thicken to a specific consistency) and a pureed diet. For some people, the dysphagia improves and they can progress to a regular diet; for others, the dysphagia is permanent. Tube feeding may become necessary in severe cases.

electrolyte balance The condition of electrolytes in the various compartments of the body (inside cells, outside cells in the blood, and the space between called interstitial fluid); electrolytes are elements or compounds that when dissolved in water dissociate into ions and can conduct an electric current. Electrolyte levels need to be in a specific balance to maintain fluid balance in the different compartments and for various metabolic functions. Two symptoms common in GI disorders, vomiting and diarrhea, can cause derangement in electrolyte balance, usually resulting in dehydration. Electrolytes include the essential minerals, sodium, potassium, phosphate, magnesium, chloride, calcium, and sulfate, in addition to organic acids, protein, and bicarbonate.

elemental formula An enteral nutrition formula containing nutrients that have been partially digested, making work easier for the intestine. Usually, this type of formula is used in GI diseases, especially those affecting the small intestine. Recent

research has shown the value of these formulas in stimulating
intestinal adaptation after resection and in inducing remission
in inflammatory bowel disease, especially when initiated as soon
as possible after surgery or disease flare-up.

emulsification The process by which an emulsifier, a compound
with a water-soluble part and a fat-soluble part, brings into
solution a fat-soluble compound. A food example is mayonnaise,
in which lecithin, an emulsifier, in the egg yolk brings together
(water-based) vinegar and oil. In the GI tract, bile acts as an
emulsifier to bring dietary fat into the watery chyme so that
fat-digesting enzymes can attack and break it down. This
function of bile, when it is absent, causes fat malabsorption.

endolumenal gastroplication A relatively new procedure for treating gastrointestinal reflux disease in which stitches are sewn near
the lower esophageal sphincter, preventing acid from the
stomach from leaking out and up into the esophagus.

endoscopy A diagnostic procedure in which a long, flexible tube
(endoscope) equipped with a fiber-optic-lighted scope is inserted
in a patient's mouth or anus to allow health care professionals
to see inside various organs (the lumen) of the digestive tract.
The endoscope enables visualization, removal and biopsy of
tissue, and the treatment of a GI bleed. From the mouth, a scope
can reach into the duodenum; from the anus a scope can reach
to the last segment of small intestine.

enteral nutrition Feeding a person by using the GI tract, which
can include eating foods, but usually means the use of tube
feeding. The tube can be inserted through the nose into the
stomach or the small intestine. Other insertion points include
surgical openings in the esophagus, stomach, or small intestine.
The formulas used can provide all the essential nutrients and
energy a person needs to survive, and such feeding can be short
term or for the rest of a person's life. Formulas are specially
designed for specific disease states, such as diabetes and kidney

disease. They can also come in forms in which the nutrients have been predigested, called *elemental formulas*, which are useful in feeding patients with various GI disorders because the GI tract does not have to work as hard as usual. In addition, the use of elemental formulas is associated with improvement in inflammatory bowel disease, possibly because of stimulation of intestinal cells to help in recovery. Some problems associated with certain methods of tube feeding include nasal and esophageal irritation, aspiration, diarrhea, fatty liver, and metabolic abnormalities.

enteritis Inflammation of the mucosal membrane of the small intestine. The cause can be bacterial, viral, or inflammatory bowel disease.

enterocolitis Inflammation of both the small intestine and the colon. The cause is often inflammatory bowel disease.

enterogastrone A hormone secreted by the intestinal mucosal cells that controls the release of chyme from the stomach into the duodenum during digestion and the release of stomach acid.

enzyme, enzyme replacement A protein produced by cells that causes a specific chemical reaction to proceed. Most enzymes are made in small quantities, but the digestive enzymes are made in large quantities. Enzyme replacements are synthetic enzymes used when a person cannot produce adequate levels of enzymes for digestion. For example, if the pancreas is damaged or diseased, it can no longer produce digestive enzymes, so enzyme replacements made of extracts from pork or beef pancreatic enzymes are taken as supplements.

epigastric The region of the abdomen in the upper zone of the stomach; usually used to refer to the location of pain, as in GI diseases.

epithelium The covering of the internal and external organs of the body. It consists of cells held together by connective material. The number of layers of cells in different locations of epithelium in the body varies. Examples include the lining of the GI tract, the respiratory tract, and blood vessels.

esophagitis Inflammation of the mucosal membrane of the esophagus. It can occur from infection, ingestion of a caustic chemical, feeding tube placement, or acid reflux from the stomach.

esophagus A cylindrical tube about 9½ inches in length through which food is conducted from the mouth to the stomach. At its base, separating it from the stomach, is the lower esophageal sphincter, which keeps the stomach's acidic contents from seeping up to the esophagus. The esophagus, like the rest of the GI tract, is characterized by layers of muscles that engage in wavelike contractions, or peristalsis, to propel food through the GI tract. The mucosal membrane of the esophagus is not equipped to handle the acid level that the stomach can, which is the reason for esophageal damage when acid refluxes up from the stomach, as in gastrointestinal reflux disease.

fat soluble The quality of a compound referring to its solubility in fat, but not water. For essential nutrients, those that are fat soluble include vitamins A, D, E, and K. They require the presence of dietary fat for absorption, and after absorption by the intestinal cells they go through the lymphatic system. The water-soluble nutrients include all the B vitamins, vitamin C, and the minerals. After absorption, the water-soluble nutrients enter the portal vein and enter the bloodstream.

fatty acid Compounds that make up dietary fat and cell membranes in the body. The body can make those compounds it needs except for two, linoleic and linolenic acid, which must be obtained through the diet. Both are abundant in vegetable oils. Fatty acids vary in the length of their chains (carbon atom chains). An intriguing area of study in GI diseases involves the short-chain fatty acids (SCFA), which appear to promote a healthy GI tract. The SCFAs are six or fewer carbons in length, and they arise in the colon from bacteria fermenting dietary fiber. Researchers believe that these compounds serve as fuel for colon cells, help prevent cancer, and promote the growth of friendly bacteria in the gut.

fecal fat test A test that measures the amount of fat in the stool to determine if malabsorption is present. Before the test, the person eats a diet containing at least 100 grams of fat per day for three days. The stool sample is then analyzed for the amount of fat excreted. Malabsorption of fat occurs in several GI diseases, such as Crohn's disease, celiac disease, and blind loop.

fiber (dietary) A complex carbohydrate the human digestive tract cannot digest, because it does not possess the enzymes to break the bonds in the molecules. The two different classes of fiber are insoluble and soluble, referring to their solubility in water. Most sources of dietary fiber—whole grains, fruits, and vegetables—contain a mix of the two types. Insoluble fiber includes cellulose, hemicellulose, and lignin. This type of fiber attracts water and holds it, much like a sponge. In the colon, this causes the stool to be larger, softer, and promotes regularity. A diet high in insoluble fiber helps prevent constipation and diverticulosis. Soluble fiber includes pectin, gum, and mucilages. This type of fiber is associated with reducing blood cholesterol and blood glucose, the latter of which is helpful for people with diabetes. In the GI tract, bacteria break down soluble fiber, producing SCFAs.

fistula An abnormal communication between two organs or tissues. Fistulae may occur anywhere, and in GI disease they may form between the intestine and the skin or some other organ. The causes include inflammatory bowel disease, cancer, and trauma. The development of a fistula as a complication of inflammatory bowel disease is serious, and increases the risk of mortality. Surgical repair is necessary but is not always successful.

flatulence Chronic intestinal gas, which can be caused by excessive motility of the GI tract, malabsorption, sudden increase in fiber intake, and eating gas-forming foods. Excessive motility of the GI tract can cause gas because most gas is normally reabsorbed by the colon. If GI tract motility is high, however, there is not enough time to adequately reabsorb the gas. Several GI disorders can cause hypermotility. Serious disease and malabsorption need to be ruled out when a person is experiencing chronic flatulence.

food additive A substance added to foods by the manufacturer for a specific function, also called *intentional additives*, to distinguish them from accidental contaminants. Some of the reasons for food additives include food preservation, color, flavor, nutrients, and texture. In GI disorders, some food additives and medication fillers can be a problem. For example, people with celiac disease must avoid gliadin/gluten, mostly found in wheat, oats, barley, and rye, for the rest of their lives. Commercial foods may contain wheat extracts as food additives for various functions. Even small amounts present only as ingredients can cause problems for people with celiac disease, so it is important to become familiar with the terms and to read labels.

food poisoning Ingestion of food contaminated with microbes from which either the microbe itself or a toxin it produces causes symptoms. Common symptoms of food poisoning are abdominal pain, nausea, fever, vomiting, and diarrhea. Although most adults recover readily from a case of food poisoning, infants, young children, the elderly, and people with compromised immune systems are at high risk for death. The most common causes of food poisoning include *Clostridium perfringens*, *Clostridium botulinum*, *Salmonella*, *Staphyloccocus aureus*, and *Listeria* monocytogenes. Experts believe that the bacteria associated with the GI diseases, peptic ulcer disease, and gastritis— *H. pylori*—can also be transmitted through foods.

fructose, fructose intolerance A simple sugar contained in fruits that is much sweeter than table sugar. Fructose intolerance is an inherited metabolic disorder that causes hypoglycemia, vomiting, lethargy, and coma. Treatment is the avoidance of fructose for the rest of the person's life.

fundoplication A surgical procedure for gastroesophageal reflux disease, in which a series of tucks are made in the fundus of the stomach around the lower esophageal sphincter. The purpose is to prevent acid from the stomach leaking into the esophagus.

galactose, galactosemia A simple sugar, differing from glucose by a slight chemical alteration. Combined with glucose, it makesup the double sugar lactose, found in milk. Galactosemia-is a disorder in which an enzyme defect makes it impossible to metabolize and use galactose as energy, resulting in a buildup of sugar levels in the blood. The disorder is genetic and causes jaundice, an enlarged liver and spleen, weight loss, diarrhea, and vomiting. In addition, if galactose is not avoided, the high blood levels cause mental retardation and the development of cataracts.

gallbladder A pear-shaped organ connected to the underside of the liver. The gallbladder receives bile synthesized by the liver via the hepatic duct. It stores and concentrates the bile, then ejects it into the cystic duct, which merges into the common bile duct leading to the duodenum. The gallbladder's ejection is stimulated by the hormone cholecystokin, which is released when fat is present in the duodenum. Bile acts as an emulsifier so that fat can be digested. Intestinal surgery can predispose a person to gallstones, and in the past it was standard practice to remove the gallbladder after intestinal resection as a preventive measure.

gastrectomy Removal of part or all of the stomach (partial or sub gastrectomy, total gastrectomy). The most common reasons for gastrectomy are ulcer and cancer. The consequences of the surgery depend on how much of the stomach was removed. The most severe problems are chronic dumping syndrome and nutritional deficiencies. The GI tract adjusts after a period of time, which varies for each individual and the type of surgery done. Many people who have had partial gastrectomy will only experience dumping syndrome initially after the surgery.

gastric Of or pertaining to the stomach.

gastric acidity Acid level of the stomach, which is dependent on the acid-secreting cells of the stomach. If the stomach's acid level is too low, several nutritional problems could develop, including protein maldigestion, and malabsorption of iron, vitamin A, and other nutrients. When the stomach secretes too much acid, however, ulcers can form in the stomach or the duodenum. Antacids counter the acidity of the stomach contents and are helpful in disorders where a lower acid level is beneficial. Several common antiulcer drugs prevent the secretion of stomach acid, but because of the importance of gastric acidity, side effects could include the problems mentioned above with low acidity.

gastric juice The secretions of the stomach cells, which include hydrochloric acid, digestive enzymes, mucus, and the intrinsic factor (needed for absorption of vitamin B_{12}).

gastric ulcer An ulcer that forms in the stomach. Acid must be present to erode the gastric mucosa, but the most common cause of gastric ulcer is *H. pylori* infection. Standard treatment is antibiotics for the eradication of the infection, antiulcer drugs to accelerate healing, and antacids to help prevent stomach pain.

gastrin Hormone secreted by the cells of the pylorus in the stomach that stimulate the parietal cells to secrete acid.

gastroesophageal reflux, gastroesophageal reflux disease Reflux of the contents of the stomach, which is acidic, into the esophagus. Reflux occurs occasionally in most people, under certain circumstances, when the lower esophageal sphincter (LES) relaxes and opens (called *heartburn*). For some people, the condition, called *gastroesophageal reflux disease* (GERD), becomes chronic. The acid from gastric contents irritates the esophagus, causing inflammation and pain. People with GERD have a higher risk for esophageal cancer than other people. Many factors can affect the lower esophageal sphincter, causing it to either open or close. Factors that cause it to relax and open include alcoholic beverages, caffeine, chocolate, cigarettes, dietary fat, mint oils, hormones released in pregnancy and in the late phase of the menstrual cycle, overeating and drinking, and many medications. Factors that cause the LES to close include dietary protein and medications. Treatment includes the avoidance of substances and foods that cause the LES to open, and the use of medications that help to keep it closed. Antacids are useful in lowering the acidity of gastric contents. If these methods fail, new surgical procedures are available.

gastrointestinal tract (GIT) The tube and all accessory structures, including the mouth, esophagus, stomach, and small and large intestine (including the anus) through which food is ingested and digested, nutrients are absorbed, and waste is excreted.

gastroparesis A condition in which the stomach becomes partially paralyzed, halting peristalsis and digestion. The cause is a localized problem with nerve impulses. This condition often occurs in diabetes because of neuropathy. Gastroparesis causes delayed gastric emptying, which in the case of diabetes worsens blood glucose control. Symptoms include nausea, vomiting, abdominal pain, and alternating constipation and diarrhea. The disorder can also promote the formation of bezoars. Treatment consists of small, frequent meals of easy-to-digest foods. If the condition becomes severe, tube feeding becomes necessary.

gastrostomy The creation of a stoma (artificial opening) from the stomach external to the body. The purpose is usually for insertion of a tube for enteral feeding. The feeding tube can deliver

nutrients either to the stomach directly or be pushed through to
the intestine into the duodenum or jejunum. A gastrostomy
may be temporary or permanent.

gliadin/gluten Gliadin is a fraction of gluten, the main protein in
wheat. Gliadin is the toxic agent that damages the small
intestine in celiac disease. Other related compounds in other
grains that cause the same reaction include hordein in barley,
secalin in rye, and avidin in oats. Treatment involves lifelong
avoidance of foods containing these compounds.

glucocorticoid A steroid hormone secreted by the adrenal glands
(located above the kidneys) with numerous effects throughout
the body, especially anti-inflammatory properties. The nutritional
effects include an increase in the production of glycogen, a
storage form of glucose. The most important of the glucocorti-
coids is cortisol. The term *corticosteroid* refers to either the
natural steroid produced by the adrenal gland or the syn-
cthetic ompound (prednisone). Prednisone is a potent anti-
inflammatory drug used in autoimmune diseases or inflammatory conditions, such as Crohn's disease or ulcerative colitis.
Serious side effects of chronic use include weight gain, muscle
wasting, high blood glucose, high blood pressure, bone deminer-
alization, and problems in all body systems.

glucose A simple sugar found in foods, especially fruits, or as part
of sucrose and lactose, the double sugars. Glucose is the principle
source of energy for the body's cells, and its level in the blood is
maintained by several homeostatic mechanisms, including the
hormone insulin. In the GI tract, carbohydrate from food is
digested to glucose, which is readily absorbed by the intestinal
cells. Protein also yields glucose, but the process takes much longer.

glutamine A nonessential amino acid that becomes important in
GI diseases and in acutely ill patients. Glutamine is the favored
energy source for the cells of the small intestine. Studies have

shown that it aids in wound healing and increases intestinal adaptation after resections. Because of its importance, glutamine is an additive in many enteral formulas.This amino acid is widely available in most foods that contain protein, and healthy people do not need to eat foods containing the amino acid. In times of acute physiologic stress and illness, however, dietary intake of glutamine is not adequate, suggesting that it is conditionally essential.

gluten-induced/sensitive enteropathy See *celiac disease*

granulomas Sandlike lesions that form in the GI tract from Crohn's disease. They can dissolve spontaneously as inflammation subsides or can become permanent. In addition, they can spread and serve as a source of infection and even gangrene.

growth hormone A hormone secreted by the pituitary gland that stimulates protein synthesis in all cells, causing growth of tissues. The specific growth effects of the hormone depend on other compounds, such as thyroid hormone, insulin, and carbohydrate. Growth hormone is considered a gut enhancer, stimulating growth of intestinal cells, especially after intestinal resections. As a gut enhancer after resections, this hormone helps the remaining small intestine to adapt and compensate in function for the lost tissue.

heartburn A painful burning sensation in the esophagus caused by reflux of acid from the stomach. See also *gastroesophageal reflux.*

Helicobacter pylori Bacteria that can inhabit the human stomach; the major cause of gastritis and peptic ulcer disease. Although a significant number of people have the infection, only about half will develop these diseases. The bacteria can be eradicated by a course of antibiotics, but the infection can be resistant in some people.

hemorrhage Loss of a significant amount of blood in a relatively short period of time. The blood loss can be due to internal bleeding or an external wound. Several GI diseases can cause hemorrhage, although slow GI bleeding is more common. Hemorrhage is a complication of peptic ulcer disease.

hiatal hernia The protrusion of the stomach through the diaphragm. The disorder is asymptomatic in most people; for others, however, symptoms include gastroesophageal reflux and difficulty breathing. Dietary approach is the same as for gastroesophageal reflux disease. If dietary changes fail to control symptoms, surgical repair may be needed.

hormone A chemical messenger made by one organ or tissue that exerts an effect in another part of the body. In the GI tract, hormones such as gastrin and enterogastrone travel in the blood from one location to produce an effect elsewhere. One example is gastrin, secreted by cells in the pyloric area of the stomach, which stimulates the release of acid from the parietal cells. Another example is enterogastrone, secreted by the intestinal cells, which travels to the stomach and causes the muscles to relax.

hyperalimentation The use of parenteral nutrition, referring to total parenteral nutrition, in which a catheter is inserted into a central blood vessel. Because hyperalimentation is placed in a central vessel, the vein can handle as many calories and nutrients as are needed for an extended period without damage to the vessel.

hyperchlorhydria Excessive gastric secretion of hydrochloric acid. Causes of exessive acid secretion can be genetic, due to stress, or a pancreatic tumor.

hypochlorhydria An abnormally low level of gastric acid secretion. Some causes include anemia, sprue, kidney disease, diabetes, gastritis, cancer, and a B vitamin deficiency.

hypoglycemia A low level of glucose in the blood, generally below 60 milligrams per deciliter of blood. In GI disease, hypoglycemia can occur as a second phase of dumping syndrome. The cause is oversecretion of insulin, which occurs because of quickly absorbed glucose from the gastric contents "dumped" into the small intestine. To prevent hypoglycemia with dumping syndrome, a diet of small frequent meals, moderate to low in carbohydrate, and an avoidance of concentrated sweets are recommended.

hypokalemia A low level of potassium in the blood. This condition can occur as a result of excessive vomiting and diarrhea, and fluid and electrolyte loss. It is dangerous, even in the short term, because it can cause heart failure.

hyponatremia A low level of sodium in the blood. This condition may be the result of excessive vomiting and diarrhea, other fluid losses, or failure of the colon to reabsorb sodium. Fluid loss and failure to reabsorb sodium can occur in colostomy and ileostomy.

iatrogenic Relating to a treatment, as in the cause of a problem. In GI disorders, iatrogenic diarrhea refers to diarrhea caused by a medication or procedure to treat disease.

ibuprofen A nonsteroidal anti-inflammatory agent also used as a pain reliever. Ibuprofen is associated with significant irritation of gastric mucosa and contributes to gastritis and peptic ulcer disease.

ileitis Inflammation of the ileum, the last segment of the small intestine; another name for Crohn's disease.

ileocecal valve The structure separating the end of the small intestine and the opening of the large intestine. The ileocecal valve controls the rate at which intestinal contents enter the colon. It is significant in intestinal surgery in that if it is removed, many medical and nutritional problems can arise, including bacterial contamination of the small intestine, increased transit time causing nutrient malabsorption, and diarrhea.

ileostomy Surgical creation of a stoma (artificial opening) from the ileum external to the body. Waste is excreted into an external appliance worn on the abdomen. Ileostomy tends to cause high electrolyte and fluid losses, as the colon is not reabsorbing fluid and minerals; consequently, stool is liquid. A low-fiber diet can help to reduce the fluid output, at least for several months after surgery. Later, fiber is gradually increased.

ileum The last segment of the small intestine. It absorbs bile salts, vitamin B_{12} and intrinsic factor, sugar, and minerals. It is the site for which Crohn's disease exhibits a predilection.

ileus Lack of movement of the GI tract. Ileus may be due to obstruction or immobility (such as after surgery). It is extremely important that a person not be fed (enterally) if ileus is present, as it could produce obstruction and perforation. Physicians will allow feeding once bowel sounds have returned, signifying normal movement.

indigestion See *dyspepsia*

inflammatory bowel disease (IBD) Severe inflammation anywhere in the GI tract, but usually in the small intestine (Crohn's disease) or large intestine (ulcerative colitis).

intestinal juice Secretions of the GI tract, including digestive enzymes, water, and mucus.

intestine The section of the GI tract that can refer to either the small intestine or the colon.

intrinsic factor A compound made by cells in the stomach that is needed for the absorption of vitamin B_{12}. Both the vitamin and the intrinsic factor leave the stomach separately, but in the low-acid environment of the intestine, they form a complex. As this complex, they are absorbed in the terminal ileum. If the terminal ileum is damaged or removed, vitamin B_{12} injections will be needed. Also, if the stomach is removed or the intrinsic factor is no longer being made at adequate levels, injections of vitamin B_{12} are needed. Even if dietary intake is adequate, without the intrinsic factor vitamin B_{12} cannot be absorbed. The disease produced by a deficiency of vitamin B_{12} is called *pernicious anemia.*

irritable bowel syndrome (IBS) A collection of symptoms that include abdominal distention, flatulence, cramps, and either constipation or diarrhea, or alternating constipation and diarrhea. IBS is not considered a disease, but it accounts for over 40 percent of visits to gastroenterologists. Treatment is to ensure adequate fluid and fiber intake, and fiber may have to be increased gradually. Medications can help with either constipation or diarrhea. IBS is not associated with any intestinal damage.

jejunostomy The creation of a stoma (artificial opening) from the jejunum external to the body. The purpose is to insert a tube for enteral feeding. The feeding tube delivers nutrients directly into the jejunum. A jejunostomy may be temporary or permanent.

jejunum The second segment of the small intestine, which is 8 feet in length and located between the duodenum and ileum. This segment of intestine absorbs the sugars glucose and galactose; amino acids and short protein chains; glycerol and fatty acids; several minerals; vitamins D, E, K, and C; most B vitamins; and alcohol.

lactose, lactose intolerance, lactase, lactase deficiency Lactose is a double sugar composed of glucose and galactose; it is found mainly in milk. To be digested, the enzyme lactase must be present in adequate amounts in the small intestine. Many people have a low level of the enzyme (lactase deficiency), which could be a result of genetics, aging, or disease affecting the enzyme-producing cells of the small intestine. In the last-mentioned instance, the problem is called secondary or functional lactose intolerance. In lactose intolerance, lactose is not degraded and therefore enters the colon intact. This causes an osmotic shift of fluid into the colon and then the bacteria ferment lactose. The resulting symptoms include bloating, cramping, nausea, gas, and diarrhea. People with lactose intolerance can avoid products containing lactose, or they can use commercial products in which the lactose has been predigested.

lactose tolerance test A test to measure blood glucose levels after ingestion of lactose (50-gram dose). If glucose only rises by 20 milligrams per deciliter or less, the test is positive for lactose intolerance. The reason for the positive result is that lactose has not been degraded into its constituents glucose and galactose, so glucose is not absorbed by the intestinal cells and does not increase appreciably in the blood.

lactulose A synthetic nonabsorbable sugar used as a laxative. Its effects are similar to lactose in the absence of lactase. Because lactulose is not degraded, it enters the colon and exerts an osmotic effect, increasing motility. Side effects may include cramping, bloating, and diarrhea. Lactulose is also used to prevent a type of coma that occurs in advanced liver disease, hepatic encephalopathy, because it reduces ammonia in the blood.

laxative See *cathartic*

linoleic acid An essential fatty acid that humans must obtain from diet. It is found in cottonseed, soybean, linseed, and safflower oils. A deficiency causes dry, scaly skin; dermatitis; hair loss; growth failure; and delayed wound healing. In people who have GI diseases that cause malabsorption of fat, a deficiency is likely. When a medium-chain triglyceride (MCT) is used as a supplement in fat malabsorption, linoleic must still be added to the diet as MCTs do not contain the fatty acid.

linolenic acid An essential fatty acid found in soybean oil and fish oils. In the body, it plays a role in immunity and growth. As with linoleic acid in fat malabsorption, linolenic must be added to the diet to prevent deficiency.

lower esophageal sphincter (LES) A sphincter that controls movement of food from the esophagus to the stomach. It is also called the cardiac sphincter. In gastroesophageal reflux disease, the LES opens when it should stay closed, allowing stomach acid to enter the esophagus and irritating the mucosal membrane. Factors that affect the pressure of the sphincter, and therefore its opening and closing, include nutrients, medications, lying down after meals, and substances such as caffeine, mint, cigarettes, alcohol, and chocolate.

lumen The interior of an organ, as in the intestinal lumen.

malabsorption A condition in which nutrients cannot be digested or absorbed and that leads to malnutrition. The most common nutrient involved in malabsorption is fat, and symptoms include cramping, bloating, and steatorrhea (fat in the stool). If fat malabsorption persists, other consequences include kidney stones, gallstones, and bone disease. Malabsorption could be caused by inadequate digestive enzymes or bile, possibly the result of inflammation or damage to the intestinal mucosa or any organ involved in digestion. Examples of GI problems that result in malabsorption include Crohn's disease, ulcerative colitis, and celiac disease.

mastication The act of chewing.

medium-chain triglycerides (MCT) A type of fat containing fatty acid chains that are six carbons or less in length. They do not require emulsification and only minimal digestive enzyme action, so they are a useful way to add energy to the diet in a person with fat malabsorption. MCTs are also useful in liver disease, because the synthesis of bile may be decreased. They can be added to enteral formulas and directly to foods.

megacolon Enlargement of the colon. Enlargement can occur in

elderly persons if they become constipated and in others who
have strictures and tumors. Megacolon can also occur in ulcerative colitis. The symptoms include abdominal distention,
flatulence, nausea, and fatigue.

melena Black, tarry stool indicative of upper GI bleeding. The
cause can be peptic ulcer disease or disease in the small intestine.

Ménétrier's disease A disease in which the gastric mucosa enlarge.
Treatment is the same as for gastritis.

metabolism The sum of all chemical changes in the body. It consists of two stages: anabolism and catabolism. Anabolism is the
synthesis of new compounds, and catabolism is the degrada-
tion of compounds.

mineral oil An intestinal irritant that produces diarrhea. It is used
as a cathartic, but it interferes with the absorption of fat-soluble
nutrients, calcium, and phosphorus.

minerals Inorganic elements, some of which are essential nutrients
and must be consumed through the diet. The major essential
minerals include calcium, phosphorus, magnesium, sulfur,
chlorine, potassium, and sodium. The trace minerals include
iron, zinc, manganese, molybdenum, copper, selenium, fluoride,
chromium, arsenic, nickel, iodine, and silicon.

nasogastric tube A thin, flexible feeding tube that is inserted
through the nose and pushed down into the stomach or the
small intestine. It cannot be used for extended periods of time
because of the irritation to nasal passages and the esophageal
mucosa.

nonsteroidal anti-inflammatory drugs (NSAIDs) Drugs used to
reduce inflammation and pain. Serious side effects include
GI bleeding, gastritis, and peptic ulcer disease.

nutrient A substance, either organic or inorganic, that the body uses
to grow or maintain tissue. The body can synthesize some
nutrients, but others must be obtained through the diet; these

nutrients are called *essential nutrients*. The six classes of nutrients are protein, fat, carbohydrate, water, vitamins, and minerals.

nutritional assessment (and nutritional status) A process by which a dietitian can determine a person's nutritional status (the state of his or her nutritional health), identify any possible risk factors that may adversely affect nutritional status, and plan nutritional intervention to correct or prevent a problem. The first step in assessment includes gathering information from the patient about current and historical dietary and nutritionally relevant lifestyle habits and reviewing physical parameters, such as blood values of various constituents, medical diagnosis, and body weight. The next step is to calculate nutrient needs, analyze the collected information, determine nutritional status, and identify any problems which preclude the person meeting nutrient needs. The last step is to plan nutritional interventions, such as a special diet, to correct current problems or prevent future problems. In GI disorders, nutritional assessment is critical because symptoms and the disease processes themselves can greatly and adversely affect nutritional status. Many interventions focus on providing nutrients in different ways, when the person cannot meet nutritional needs by eating foods.

obstruction In GI disease, a blockage at some location in the GI tract. A blockage can occur anywhere, but it is most common in the intestines. The cause could be a tumor or cancerous growth, active inflammation, or the formation of scar tissue.

occult blood Blood found by microscopic examination or chemical analysis that is not visible to the naked eye. People with GI problems often have occult blood in their stool.

oligosaccharide Carbohydrates of two to ten carbon atoms, including sucrose (table sugar), lactose (milk sugar), and two indigestible forms (stachyose and raffinose). These last two forms are also classed as fructooligosaccharides and are found in plant products. Because of their indigestibility, oligosaccharides enter the colon intact where colonic bacteria ferment them, causing flatulence.

osmosis, osmotic pressure Osmosis is a universal law, like gravity, that occurs when the liquid part of a solution passes through a semipermeable membrane from the side of lower concentration to the side of higher concentration, equalizing the concentration of the solution on either side of the membrane. Osmotic pressure refers to the drawing force of substances dissolved in solution; it is the force exerted by the substances on the solvent, causing it to pass through the membrane and equalize concentration. The significance of osmosis in GI disease relates to the intestinal membrane and the lumen of the organ. The intestinal membrane acts as a semipermeable membrane so that if an osmotically active substance, such as intact lactose, enters the intestine, it exerts osmotic pressure to shift fluid from surrounding tissues into the intestinal lumen. The effects of this pressure as fluid fills the intestine include abdominal cramping, distention, nausea, gas, and diarrhea. Osmosis is the mechanism of lactose intolerance and the use of laxatives such as saline cathartics; both produce osmotic diarrhea.

osteomalacia Adult rickets, in which bones soften because of a lack of calcium, phophorus, or vitamin D. It is different from osteoporosis, in which bones demineralize but become brittle instead of soft. Osteomalacia is one form of bone disease that can arise from GI disorders that produce fat malabsorption because calcium forms soaps with undigested fat and is pulled out of the intestine before it can be absorbed. Also, fat malabsorption causes fat-soluble vitamins (one of which is vitamin D) to not be absorbed.

ostomy A surgical procedure that involves the creation of a stoma (artificial opening) in the wall of the abdomen. The purpose of an ostomy can be for the placement of a feeding tube or to allow for excretion of stool if the colon or rectum and anus have been removed because of disease. Diseases that commonly require ostomies include Crohn's disease, ulcerative colitis, and intestinal cancer. Depending on the location of the ostomy (ileostomy or colostomy), severe nutritional problems can arise.

oxalate A compound found in plants that forms an unabsorbable complex with essential minerals, such as calcium. This complex is excreted, wasting calcium and also increasing the risk for kidney stones. Foods high in oxalate include spinach, rhubarb, beets, berries, plums, and tea. Oxalate becomes a problem for people with GI diseases that cause fat malabsorption, making them susceptible to kidney stones, gallstones, and bone disease because of calcium depletion. People who have fat malabsorption, especially if it is chronic, should follow a low-oxalate diet.

pancreas, pancreatic juice The pancreas is an organ cradled in the duodenum and connected to that segment of small intestine by the pancreatic duct, which merges into the common bile duct. It is important in digestion because its cells produce pancreatic juice containing digestive enzymes, electrolytes, and bicarbonate. As the pancreas secretes its juice into the duodenum, bicarbonate reduces the acidity of the chyme that came from the acidic stomach. This process is important for two reasons: the duodenum would be damaged by the high acid, and intestinal enzymes are active at a lower acid environment than are gastric enzymes. The pancreas is also the site of insulin and glucagon, two hormones that regulate blood glucose. Any problem arising in the pancreas or its duct will adversely affect digestion and nutrient absorption. In that event, special enzyme replacement supplements are available to partially replace the enzymes from the pancreas.

parenteral nutrition A method of providing nutrition in which a solution containing essential nutrients is delivered directly into the bloodstream. The two main types of parenteral nutrition are peripheral parenteral nutrition (PPN) and central or total parenteral nutrition (CPN or TPN). With PPN, the catheter (needle connected to a nutrient solution bag) is placed in a blood vessel in an arm or leg. With TPN, the catheter is inserted into a central vessel such as the superior or inferior vena cava, or jugular vein. When possible, it is preferable to use PPN because of less risk involved in catheter placement. In TPN, the needle can puncture a lung or the heart. If the person will need parenteral nutrition for a significant length of time, TPN is used because the large blood vessel can better withstand the solution than can a smaller, peripheral vessel. Another reason for using TPN is if the person needs a solution containing a high level of energy and nutrients; a highly concentrated solution could damage a smaller, peripheral blood vessel. In GI disease, because the GI tract may not be functioning, it is often necessary to use parenteral nutrition.

parietal cell Cells in the stomach that produce hydrochloric acid and the intrinsic factor.

pepsin A protein-digesting enzyme made by the stomach. When secreted, it is in an inactive form, pepsinogen, which becomes activated by the presence of hydrochloric acid.

peptic ulcer disease (PUD) The presence of circumscribed areas of erosion in either the stomach or the duodenum, caused by acid. Although acid is a direct cause of the erosion and must be present for it to occur, other factors affect PUD development. Chief of these is the bacteria *H. pylori*. Other contributing factors include chronic use of nonsteroidal anti-inflammatory drugs and other medications that irritate the gastric mucosa, alcohol abuse, excessive secretion of gastric acid, and weakened defenses.

peritonitis Inflammation of the peritoneum, the membrane covering the abdominal wall and the organs. The cause of peritonitis is often an infection, but it could be an irritating agent. Many GI diseases can cause peritonitis, as can rupture of the appendix. Signs and symptoms of peritonitis include abdominal distention and tenderness, pain, vomiting, absence of bowel sounds, fever and chills, inability to defecate, and labored breathing. Treatment consists of antibiotics and enemas, and may require a rectal tube to evacuate stool.

phenolphthalein A laxative that irritates the intestinal mucosa and stimulates motility. Side effects include potassium depletion, malabsorption of vitamin D, glucose, calcium, and other minerals.

protein Organic compounds essential for all living organisms. Proteins consist of specific sequences of amino acids that form various shapes. The shapes of proteins give rise to specific functions in the body. Protein is used to make cells, enzymes, hormones, and antibodies, and it can be oxidized for energy if needed. Food sources of protein vary in their quality, a measure of the amount of essential amino acids. High-quality protein sources include meat, dairy products, and eggs. Plant proteins are generally lower in quality, but soybeans contain good quality protein. Plant sources include legumes and grains. In GI disease, protein may be lost whenever malabsorption occurs or when intestinal tissue is inflamed, bleeding, or damaged. Blood loss from the upper or lower GI also depletes protein. The normal protein need is 0.8 gram per kilogram of body weight (not including excessive body fat). In malabsorption, inflammatory bowel disease, or other GI disease, protein need may be higher.

protein-losing enteropathy A condition in which protein is lost because of disease. Diseases that tend to cause protein loss include Crohn's disease, ulcerative colitis, and celiac disease.

pureed diet A diet composed of foods that have been blended and strained and are almost liquid in consistency. Pureed foods

require no chewing and are generally easier to swallow than
whole foods, so the diet is used with people who have dentition
or swallowing problems.

pylorus, pyloric, pyloric sphincter The tubular lower portion of
the stomach that angles to the right of the body of the stomach
toward the duodenum. The pyloric sphincter controls the rate
at which partially digested food (chyme) leaves the stomach and
enters the duodenum.

radionuclide An isotope that undergoes radioactive decay (isotopes of iodine, cobalt, phosphorus, and other elements) used
in diagnostic procedures to provide imaging of internal parts
of the body. Also used in treating cancer.

raffinose A carbohydrate (fructooligosaccharide) contained in
beets, underground roots and stems, and molasses. It is partially
digested in the human GI tract, but colon bacteria ferment
most of the compound.

ranitidine An antiulcer drug that reduces gastric acid secretion.
Side effects include reduced iron and vitamin B_{12} absorption,
GI bleeding, and vitamin K deficiency.

rectum The last portion of the colon, about 4¾ inches in length,
which ends in the anal canal. The anus, the opening of the anal
canal that is external to the body, is guarded by sphincters.

reflux esophagitis see *gastroesophageal reflux disease*

regurgitation Backward flow from the normal direction, as in
swallowed food returning into the mouth.

resection, bowel Surgical procedure involving removal of a portion
of the intestine and reconnecting the two segments on either
side of the portion excised.

residue The components of food remaining that enter the colon
after digestion and absorption in the small intestine. Most of the
residue consists of dietary fiber from plant materials, but
it may include connective tissue from tough cuts of meat or

parts of poultry skin. A low-residue diet is often prescribed for the relief of diarrhea. It differs from a low-fiber diet only in avoiding tough meat, poultry skin, and lactose, which is often a problem in diarrhea.

saliva, salivary amylase Saliva is the secretion from the salivary glands, containing mainly salivary amylase, the enzyme to begin some starch digestion. Saliva is also important in helping liquefy foods, making chewing and swallowing easier. Many medications can cause a reduction in saliva, causing dry mouth. Such a reduction can cause problems especially for the elderly, who are prone to reduced saliva levels, and may adversely affect food intake.

senna A compound that is an intestinal irritant, and is often used as a laxative. Senna is found in the leaves of *Cassia angustifolia* and is used in commercial laxative preparations. Side effects include potassium depletion and malabsorption.

short bowel syndrome (SBS) A condition caused by removal of portions of the intestine. It causes nutrient malabsorption, diarrhea, bone disease, and other GI problems. Severity depends on many factors, but mostly on the amount of the intestine removed. Treatment focuses on a staged approach for diet, beginning first with parenteral nutrition and enteral nutrition using elemental formulas. The diet progresses to combinations of these feeding methods and gradual weaning from them, as regular foods are gradually reintroduced.

short-chain fatty acid (SCFA) Fatty acids consisting of six or fewer carbons; colonic bacteria ferment soluble fiber and produce SCFAs. SCFAs have several beneficial effects in the colon, including increasing acidity of the colon, limiting colon cells' absorption of ammonia (a toxin), and promoting bacterial growth in the colon. These effects are thought to lower the risk of colon cancer. These fatty acids also serve as an energy source for colon cells and in short bowel syndrome may provide a significant source of total energy. SCFAs have been used as enema additives in the treatment of ulcerative colitis.

small intestine The part of the GI tract that consists of three segments: duodenum, jejunum, and ileum. The small intestine is about 21 feet in length, with an average diameter of 2½ inches. It is the site of most digestion and virtually all nutrient absorption. It lies between the stomach and the large intestine.

soft diet A diet that can either be used for chewing problems (mechanical soft) or as a transition diet in illness, especially GI disorders (GI soft). It consists of foods that are soft in texture, with no tough or fibrous parts, and that are prepared without the use of spices. The specifics of the diet vary from one institution to another.

sprue (tropical) A disease causing significant malabsorption that is common in tropical and subtropical regions. The exact cause is unknown but is probably a combination of inadequate nutrition and chronic infection. It is different from celiac disease (nontropical sprue), in which gluten acts as a toxin in the small intestine, causing severe damage.

stachyose A fructooligosaccharide contained in legumes and beets that is mostly indigestible. It is fermented in the colon by bacteria and often causes flatulence.

steatorrhea A type of diarrhea caused by the malabsorption of fat. The stool is foamy and greasy, indicating the presence of undigested fat. Steatorrhea accompanies several GI diseases that cause fat malabsorption. Consequences of chronic or severe steatorrhea include loss of energy, loss of fat-soluble nutrients, kidney stones and gallstones, and bone disease. It is usually treated with a low-fat diet, but the cause must be determined and treated as well.

stoma Artificial opening external to the body created for either placement of a feeding tube or excretion of waste. See also *ostomy*.

stricture In GI disease, a narrowing of a section of intestine usually caused by scar tissue formation. It is a common complication of Crohn's disease and causes intestinal obstruction.

sucrose, sucrose intolerance Sucrose, often called table sugar, is a double sugar and is made from cane or beet sugar. A person who does not have adequate amounts of the enzyme sucrase is sucrose intolerant. The condition is similar to lactose intolerance in that sucrose will enter the colon intact, causing diarrhea and other GI symptoms because of osmotic pressure. The dietary approach is to avoid sucrose.

sulfonamides, sulfasalazine Drugs used to treat infections and also used chronically in inflammatory bowel disease to prevent flare-ups. They interfere with folate, vitamins C and K, and protein metabolism. Side effects include anorexia, nausea, vomiting, and diarrhea.

trigylceride Dietary fat consisting of three fatty acids attached to a glycerol backbone and the main storage form of fat in the body. The fatty acids vary in length and number of double bonds, which gives rise to different fats with varying properties: polyunsaturated fats, monounsaturated fat, and saturated fat. The different types of fat have many health implications, with saturated fat raising blood cholesterol.

trypsin A protein-digesting enzyme made and secreted by the pancreas. The pancreas secretes the enzyme in an inactive form, which becomes activated when it reaches the duodenum.

ulcerative colitis One of the two types of inflammatory bowel disease, involving inflammation and bleeding of the colon. The sections of the colon most commonly affected are the sigmoid colon and rectum. The cause of the disease is unknown, but is now believed to be autoimmune in nature. It is characterized by flare-ups and remissions. Symptoms include severe and sometimes bloody diarrhea, abdominal cramping and pain, and fever. A patient with ulcerative colitis may lose weight and develop nutritional anemias, although nutrient malabsorption is not direct because the small intestine is not affected. The disease increases the risk of cancer and often necessitates colectomy and a resulting colostomy.

vagotomy, truncal vagotomy, vagus nerve A surgical procedure used to treat peptic ulcer disease in which the vagus nerve is severed. The purpose is to reduce gastric acid secretion, as the vagus nerve stimulates this secretion.

villi Fingerlike projections that sit on the folds of the small intestine, around which reside the intestinal mucosal cells. The villi and the intestinal folds effectively increase the surface area of the small intestine. The increased surface area is critical in providing a larger area for the absorption of nutrients. In some GI diseases, the villi become flattened, reducing their absorptive area and causing nutrient malabsorption and malnutrition. When a person is fed parenterally, the villi tend to flatten and atrophy.

vitamin B$_{12}$ A water-soluble B vitamin (also called *cobalamin*) found in animal products, especially milk and dairy products. Its chief functions are making new cells and maintaining the nervous system. Deficiency symptoms include anemia (pernicious anemia), fatigue, paralysis, skin abnormalities, and tongue abnormalities. Strict vegetarians are at risk for a deficiency, as are people with various GI diseases. Gastrectomy can cause deficiency because of removal of cells that produce the intrinsic factor. Lower GI diseases that strike the terminal ileum, such as Crohn's disease and celiac disease, can also cause deficiency because the vitamin is absorbed there. Blind loop syndrome can cause deficiency because the bacteria use up the vitamin; short bowel syndrome can cause the deficiency because of bacterial overgrowth or removal of the terminal ileum.

whey The liquid that remains after curd and cream are separated from coagulated milk. The protein in whey is isolated and added to reduced-fat versions of foods such as hamburgers or cheesecake, replacing their traditional high-fat counterparts. It contains most of the lactose from the original milk, little protein, and no fat. Because of its lactose content, whey is avoided by people with lactose intolerance.

Zollinger-Ellison syndrome A tumor of the pancreas that causes excessive secretion of gastric acid producing ulceration of the esophagus, stomach, and duodenum. Symptoms include malabsorption and diarrhea. It is important to distinguish this disorder from peptic ulcer disease.

References

■ · · · · · · ■

BENINI, L. ET AL. 1994. "Gastric Emptying of Solids Is Markedly Delayed When Meals are Fried." *Digestive Diseases and Sciences* 39(11): 2288–94.

BISCHOFF, S. C. ET AL. 1996. "Prevalence of Adverse Reactions to Food in Patients with Gastrointestinal Disease." *Allergy* 51: 811.

D'ARGENIO, G., and G. MAZZACCA. 1999. "Short-Chain Fatty Acid in the Human Colon: Relation to Inflammatory Bowel Diseases and Colon Can cer." *Advances in Experimental Medicine and Biology* 472: 149–58.

DIELEMAN, L. A., and W. D. HEIZER. 1998. "Nutritional Issues in Inflamma-tory Bowel Disease." *Gastroenterology Clinics of North America* 27(2): 435–5.

DOUGHTY, D. B., and D. B. JACKSON. 1993. *Gastrointestinal Disorders.* St. Louis: Mosby.

DROSSMAN, D. A. ET AL. 1997. "Irritable Bowel Syndrome: A Technical Review for Practice Guideline Development." *Gastroenterology* 112: 2120.

EL-ZAATARI, F. A. ET AL. 1999. "Characterization of *Mycobacterium paratu berculosis* p36 Antigen and Its Seroreactivities in Crohn's Disease." *Cur rent Issues in Intestinal Microbiology* 39(2): 115–19.

ESCOTT-STUMP, S. 1997. *Nutrition and Diagnosis-Related Care.* Baltimore: Williams and Wilkins.

GALMICHE, J. P. 1998. "Gastro-Oesophageal Reflux: Does it Matter What You Eat? *Gut* 42: 318–19.

GISBERT, J. P., J. M. PAJARES, and C. LOSA. "*Helicobacter pylori* and Gastro-esophageal Reflux Disease: Friends or Foes." *Hepto-Gastroenterolgy* 1023–29.

GOLDSTEIN, N. S. ET AL. 1997. "Crohn's-Like Complications in Patients with Ulcerative Colitis After Total Proctocolectomy and Ileal Pouch-Anal Anastomosis." *American Journal of Surgical Pathology* 21: 1343.

GOUTTEBEL, M. C. ET AL. 1992. "Influence of n-Acetylglutamine or Gluta-mine Infusion on Plasma Amino Acid Concentrations During the Early Phase of Small Bowel Adaptation in the Dog." *Journal of Parenteral and Enteral Nutrition.* 16:117–21

HOLLOWAY, R. H. ET AL. 1997. "Effect of Intraduodenal Fat on Lower Oesophageal Sphincter Function and Gastro-Oesophageal Reflux." *Gut* 40: 449–53.

HOLTMANN, G., C. CAIN, and P. MALFERTHEINER. 1999. "Gastric *Helicobacter pylori* Infection Accelerates Healing of Reflux Esophagitis During Treatment with the Proton Pump Inhibitor Pantoprazole." *Gastroenterology* 117: 11–16.

KENNEDY, M. V., and E. J. ZARLING. 1998. "Answers to 10 Key Questions on Diverticular Disease of the Colon." *Comprehensive Therapy* 24(8): 364–69.

KJELLIN, A. ET AL. 1996. "Gastroesophageal Reflux in Obese Patients Is Not Reduced by Weight Reduction." *Scandinavian Journal of Gastroenterology* 31(11): 1047–51.

KOHLER, L., S. SAUERLAND, and E. NEUGEBAUER. 1999. "Diagnosis and Treatment of Diverticular Disease: Results of a Consensus Development Conference. The Scientific Committee of the European Association for Endoscopic Surgery." *Surgical Endoscopy* 13(4) (): 430–36.

MAHAN, L., KATHLEEN, and S. ESCOTT-STUMP, 1999, 2000. *Krause's Food, Nutrition, and Diet Therapy*, 10th ed. Philadelphia: Saunders, 1999.

MARSHALL, B. J. "*Helicobacter pylori:* A Primer for 1994." *Gastroenterologist* 1(4) (1993): 241–47.

McNAMARA, D., and C. O'MORAIN. 1999. "Gastroesophageal Reflux Disease and *Helicobacter pylori:* An Intricate Relation." *Gut* 45(suppl 1): 113–17.

Merck Manual of Medical Information—Home Edition CD-ROM. 1999. McGraw-Hill Professions Division.

Mosby's Medical, Nursing, and Allied Health Dictionary, 4th ed. 1994. St. Louis: Mosby.

MURRAY, J. A. 1999. "The Widening Spectrum of Celiac Disease." *American Journal of Clinical Nutrition* 69: 354–65.

NORDGAARD, I., B. S. HANSEN, and P. B. MORTENSEN. 1996. "Importance of Colonic Support for Energy Absorption as Small Bowel Failure Proceeds." *American Journal of Clinical Nutrition* 64: 222–31.

PAGANA, K. D., and T. J. PAGANA. 1998. *Mosby's Manual of Diagnostic and Laboratory Tests.* St. Louis: Mosby.

PENAGINI, R., M. MANGANO, and P. A. BIANCHI. 1998. "Effect of Increasing the Fat Content But Not the Energy Load of a Meal on Gastro-Eesophageal Reflux and Lower Oesophageal Sphincter Motor Function." *Gut* 42: 330–33.

PENNINGTON, J. 1998. *A. T. Bowes and Church's Food Values of Portions Commonly Used*. Philadelphia: Lippincott.

Recommended Dietary Allowances, 10th ed. 1989. Washington, D. C.: National Academy Press,

RUHL, C. E., and J. E. EVERHART. October 1999. "Overweight, But Not High Dietary Fat Intake, Increases Risk of Gastroesophageal Reflux Disease Hospitalization: The NHANES I Epidemiologic Followup Study. First National Health and Nutrition Examination Survey." *Annals of Epidemiology* 9(7): 424–35.

Saunders Drug Handbook for Health Professionals 2000. 2000. Philadelphia: Saunders.

SHAKER, J. L. ET AL. 1997. "Hypocalcemia and Skeletal Disease as Present ing Features of Celiac Disease." *Archives of Internal Medicine* 157(9): 1013–16

SHILS, M. E., J. A. OLSON, and M. SHIKE. 1994. *Modern Nutrition in Health and Disease*. Philadelphia: Lea and Febiger.

SHODA, R. ET AL. 1996. "Epidemiologic Analysis of Crohn's Disease in Japan: Increased Dietary Intake of n-6 Polyunsaturated Fatty Acids and Animal Protein Relates to Increased Incidence of Crohn's Disease in Japan." *American Journal of Clinical Nutrition* 63: 741

SPELLET, G. 1994. "Nutritional Management of Common Gastrointestinal Problems." *Nurse Practitioner Forum* 5: 24.

STROCCHI, A. and M. D. LEVITT. 1998. "Intestinal Gas." In *Gastrointestinal and Liver Disease*, 6th ed., edited by M. Feldman, M. H. Sleisenger, and B. F. Scharschmidt. Philadelphia: Saunders.

Surgeon General's Report on Nutrition and Health. 1988. Washington, D. C.: U. S. Government Printing Office.

WHITNEY, E. N., C. B. CATALDO, and S. R. ROLFES. 1998. *Understanding Normal and Clinical Nutrition*. Belmont, Calif.: Wadsworth.

WILSON, L. J., W. MA, and B. I. HIRSCHOWITZ. October 1999. "Association of Obesity with Hiatal Hernia and Esophagitis." *American Journal of Gastroenterology*. 94(10): 2840–44.

ZEMAN, F. J., and D. M. NEY. 1996. *Applications in Medical Nutrition Therapy*. Upper Saddle River, N.J.: Prentice Hall, .

Index

■　·　·　·　·　·　■

Gastrointestinal
Disorders
and
Nutrition

Also by Tonia Reinhard, M. S., R. D.

The Vitamin Sourcebook